PANCE/PANRE Challenge

Eve B. Hoover, DMSc, PA-C, DFAAPA, is an Associate Professor at Midwestern University. She received her Physician Assistant (PA) education from Saint Louis University, followed by a master's degree in Advanced Physician Assistant Studies focused on Education and Leadership from A.T. Still University. She then earned a Doctor of Medical Science in PA Education from the University of Lynchburg. Eve has been recognized as a Distinguished Fellow of the American Academy of Physician Assistants for commitment to medical practice, service and leadership within the PA profession. Eve has published peer-reviewed manuscripts on topics such as Travel Medicine, Infectious Disease, Orthopedics and medical practice and is also a peer reviewer for the journal *Clinician Reviews*. Eve entered PA education after fifteen years of practice in a variety of primary care settings. Eve completed a postgraduate academic fellowship at Midwestern University and then joined the didactic team as an Assistant Professor. Eve has presented at state, regional, and national venues on topics related to PA practice and PA education. She is an active member of Physician Assistant Education Association (PAEA). She enjoys the opportunity to teach students and clinicians about areas of medicine including but not limited to HEENT, dermatology, rheumatology, infectious disease, gastroenterology, urology, neurology, pediatrics, endocrinology, ethics, laboratory assessment, history and physical exam and clinician wellness. She serves as one of the Midwestern University PA Program Challenge Bowl faculty advisors and has been active in question development to support student learning for years. Eve also serves on the CME committee for the Arizona State Association of Physician Assistants and is committed to providing relevant, effective, comprehensive learning opportunities for students and clinicians and is a member of the PAEA (Physician Assistant Education Association).

Kimberly A. Carter, DMSc, PA-C, RD, is an Associate Professor and Clinical Coordinator with Midwestern University's PA Program. Kimberly completed a Dietetic Internship at Johns Hopkins Bayview Medical Center and practiced inpatient nutrition and dietetics before transitioning into medicine. She earned her Master's degree in Physician Assistant Studies from A.T. Still University and Doctor of Medical Science in PA Education from the University of Lynchburg. Her clinical experience is within the fields of Geriatrics, Internal Medicine, and Gastroenterology. Kimberly has published a peer-reviewed manuscript on curriculum development and is also a peer reviewer for the journal of *Clinical Advisor* and is a member of the PAEA (Physician Assistant Education Association). Kimberly instructs on a variety of medical subjects including but not limited to nutrition, gastroenterology, nephrology, urology, acid-base disorders, electrolyte abnormalities, physical diagnosis, clinical laboratory and diagnostic medicine, health maintenance and preventative wellness, and pharmacology. Kimberly facilitates small group activities across the clinical medicine curriculum and serves as a co-faculty advisor for the Midwestern University PA program Challenge Bowl Team. She is involved in the assessment of student learning and contributes to test-item writing for formative and summative exams. Kimberly aims to develop authentic assessments to support the attainment of competency and readiness for clinical practice. Aside from her academic and clinic roles, she enjoys presenting at state and national conferences on CME content.

Robyn A. Sears, DMSc, PA-C, is an Associate Professor at Midwestern University. She received her undergraduate degree from the University of Minnesota in the field of Microbiology. She attended A.T. Still University's PA Program, earning her MS in Physician Assistant Studies and went on to complete her Doctor of Medical Science degree with a concentration in education and leadership at the University of Lynchburg. Robyn practiced clinically as a PA for 18 years in the areas of emergency medicine and interventional pain management before transitioning to PA education in June of 2015. She lectures on topics to include HEENT, ophthalmology, infectious disease, radiology, neurology, musculoskeletal, emergency medicine, gastroenterology, and professionalism. She is an active member of Physician Assistant Education Association (PAEA). Robyn has presented nationally, regionally, and at the state levels on topics related to patient care and professionalism. She has been published in the peer-reviewed *Journal of the American Academy of Physician Assistants* on acute cancer pain management and is a peer reviewer for the journal. Robyn serves on the Awards Committee and the CME committee for the Arizona State Association of Physician Assistants and prepares and revises questions for the state Challenge Bowl.

Sarah L. Bolander, DMSc, PA-C, DFAAPA, is an Associate Professor in the PA program at Midwestern University and Adjunct Faculty in the Doctor of Medical Science (DMSc) program at the University of Lynchburg. She is a graduate of both of these programs earning her Master of Medical Science Degree at Midwestern and her DMSc Degree with a focus in PA education at University of Lynchburg. At Midwestern University, she lectures on topics including dermatology, orthopaedics, pediatrics, surgery, pulmonary, endocrine, neurology, imaging, procedural skills, and evidence-based medicine. Sarah continues to work clinically in orthopaedic surgery at Cactus Pediatric Orthopaedics. Sarah is a Distinguished Fellow with the American Academy of Physician Assistants (AAPA) and an active member of Physician Assistant Education Association (PAEA), Arizona State Association of Physician Assistants (ASAPA), and Physician Assistants in Orthopaedic Surgery (PAOS). Sarah serves her profession both locally and nationally. She is the 2021–2022 ASAPA President and an Arizona Representative for the AAPA House of Delegates since 2018. She serves on the Education Steering Committee for PAEA and is the Conference Workshop Lead for PAOS where she also routinely provides Self-Assessment Questions for CME events. Sarah has the privilege of presenting regularly at local, regional, and national conferences. She has written a book chapter and is published in several peer-reviewed medical journals.

PANCE/PANRE Challenge Quick Q&A Review

Eve B. Hoover, DMSc, PA-C, DFAAPA

Kimberly A. Carter, DMSc, PA-C, RD

Robyn A. Sears, DMSc, PA-C

Sarah L. Bolander, DMSc, PA-C, DFAAPA

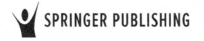

SPRINGER PUBLISHING

Image Credits (By Chapter and Question/Answer Number): **CHAPTER 1:** 28. Courtesy of James Heilman. 64 and 93. Knechtel, Maureen A. (2020) *EKGs for the Nurse Practitioner and Physician Assistant*, 3rd ed. Springer Publishing Company. **CHAPTER 2:** 8. Courtesy of Julia/Wikimedia. 16. Courtesy of Jared Heaton, D.O. 24 and 44. Courtesy of Sarah L. Bolander, DMSc, PA-C, DFAAPA. **CHAPTER 3:** 6. Courtesy of Klaus D. Peter. 34. Myrick, K., Karosas, L. (2019). *Advanced Health Assessment and Differential Diagnosis: Essentials for Clinical Practice*. Springer Publishing Company. 60. Courtesy of Philippe Chanson and Sylvie Salenave. **CHAPTER 4:** 6 and 15. Courtesy of Eugenia P. Roberts, DDS. 24. Courtesy of Sarah L. Bolander, DMSc, PA-C, DFAAPA. **CHAPTER 8:** 15. Courtesy of WeisSagung. 37. Courtesy of Velika Lotwala and Sarah L. Bolander, DMSc, PA-C, DFAAPA. **CHAPTER 9:** 5. Courtesy of GE Malone. 15. Courtesy of Sarah L. Bolander, DMSc, PA-C, DFAAPA. 32. Courtesy of Rylan East, MMS, and Sarah L. Bolander, DMSc, PA-C, DFAAPA. 47. Campo, T. M. *Medical Imaging for the Health Care Provider*. 2016, Springer Publishing Company. **CHAPTER 12:** 16 and 54. Campo, T. M. (2016). *Medical Imaging for the Health Care Provider*. Springer Publishing Company. 67. Courtesy of James Heilman. 77. Clinical Cases. Wikimedia Commons. **CHAPTER 13:** 36. Wikimedia Commons. **CHAPTER 14:** 24. Gawlik, K. S., Melnyk, B. M., Teall, A. M. (2021). *Evidence-Based Physical Examination: Best Practices for Health and Well-Being Assessment*. Springer Publishing Company.

Springer Publishing Company, LLC
11 West 42nd Street, New York, NY 10036
www.springerpub.com
examprepconnect.springerpub.com/

Acquisitions Editor: Suzanne Toppy
Compositor: Integra

ISBN: 9780826158628
ebook ISBN: 9780826158635
DOI: 10.1891/9780826158635

21 22 23 24 / 5 4 3 2 1

The author and the publisher of this Work have made every effort to use sources believed to be reliable to provide information that is accurate and compatible with the standards generally accepted at the time of publication. Because medical science is continually advancing, our knowledge base continues to expand. Therefore, as new information becomes available, changes in procedures become necessary. We recommend that the reader always consult current research and specific institutional policies before performing any clinical procedure or delivering any medication. The author and publisher shall not be liable for any special, consequential, or exemplary damages resulting, in whole or in part, from the readers' use of, or reliance on, the information contained in this book. The publisher has no responsibility for the persistence or accuracy of URLs for external or third-party Internet websites referred to in this publication and does not guarantee that any content on such websites is, or will remain, accurate or appropriate.

LCCN: 2021915630

Contact sales@springerpub.com to receive discount rates on bulk purchases.

Publisher's Note: **New and used products purchased from third-party sellers are not guaranteed for quality, authenticity, or access to any included digital components.**

Printed in the United States of America.

We would like to dedicate this book to the thousands of patients we have been privileged to care for, hundreds of students that inspire us daily, and countless numbers of PAs and other healthcare providers who have been mentors, colleagues, and friends. We want to thank our families for their enthusiastic support and unwavering encouragement during the development of this book. Our families consistently champion our efforts to advance PA education and growth of our profession.

Contents

Reviewers   *xiii*
Foreword   *xv*
Preface   *xvii*
Pass Guarantee   *xix*
Introduction   *xxi*

Chapter 1: Cardiovascular System   *1*

Chapter 2: Dermatologic System   *29*

Chapter 3: Endocrine System   *43*

Chapter 4: Eyes, Ears, Nose, and Throat   *61*

Chapter 5: Gastrointestinal System/Nutrition   *79*

Chapter 6: Genitourinary System (Male and Female)   *101*

Chapter 7: Hematologic System   *113*

Chapter 8: Infectious Diseases   *125*

Chapter 9: Musculoskeletal System   *139*

Chapter 10: Neurologic System   *159*

Chapter 11: Psychiatry/Behavioral Science   *175*

Chapter 12: Pulmonary System   *191*

Chapter 13: Renal System   *213*

Chapter 14: Reproductive System (Male and Female)   *227*

Chapter 15: Professional Practice   *243*

Index   *251*

Reviewers

Shailja Amin, PA-C, Physician Assistant, Immuno-Oncology, Phoenix, Arizona

Adrijana Anderson, MMS, PA-C, Physician Assistant, Critical Care and Hospital Internal Medicine, Mayo Clinic Arizona, Phoenix, Arizona

Edward Bermingham, MMS, PA-C, Adjunct Professor, Physician Assistant Program, Midwestern University College of Health Sciences, Glendale, Arizona

Kari Bernard, PhD, PA-C, Associate Director of Research and Capstone Activities, AT Still University-Arizona School of Health Sciences Doctor of Medical Science program, Psychiatric Physician Assistant, Orion Behavioral Health Network

Rachel Byrne, MS PA-C, Faculty Instructor, University of Colorado Child Health Associate/Physician Assistant Program, Aurora, Colorado

Robyn L. Chalupa, DSc, PA-C, Chair, Doctorate in Physician Assistant Studies in Orthopaedics, US Army-Baylor University, Waco, Texas

Bettie Coplan, PhD, PA-C, Assistant Professor, Department of Physician Assistant Studies, Northern Arizona University, Flagstaff, Arizona

Carrlene Donald, MMS, PA-C, Assistant Professor in Otolaryngology, Mayo Clinic College of Medicine and Science, Phoenix, Arizona

Tanya L. Fernandez, MS, PA-C, IBCLC, Assistant Professor, University of Colorado Child Health Associate/Physician Assistant Program, Aurora, Colorado

Sarah Gerber, MMS, PA-C, CPAAPA, Certified Physician Assistant, Phoenix West Internal Medicine, Adjunct Assistant Professor, Physician Assistant Program, Midwestern University College of Health Sciences, Glendale, Arizona

Nicholas Goodman, MMS, PA-C, Physician Assistant, Phoenix Pediatrics, Ltd., Adjunct Faculty, Physician Assistant Program, Midwestern University College of Health Sciences, Glendale, Arizona

Rebekah Hudson, MPAS, PA-C, Emergency Medicine Physician Assistant, Director of Physician Assistant Emergency Medicine Post Graduate Fellowship, University of Missouri Hospital, Columbia, Missouri

Stephanie Jalaba, MMS, PA-C, Assistant Professor, Department of PA Medicine, Michigan State University College of Osteopathic Medicine, East Lansing, Michigan

Cathy Kelley, PA-C, Physician Assistant/Child Health Associate, Pediatrix, Phoenix, Arizona

Shuli Leiken, MMS, PA-C, Surgical Physician Assistant, Bloomington, Illinois

Susan LeLacheur, DrPH, PA-C, Professor of Physician Assistant Studies, The George Washington University School of Medicine and Health Sciences, Washington, DC

Velika Lotwala, PA-C, Diplomate Fellow, SDPA, Physician Assistant, Epiphany Dermatology, Peoria, Arizona

Bryan Nelson, DMSc, PA-C, Principle Instructor, Physician Assistant Program, Rocky Mountain University of Health Professions, Provo, Utah

Kaycee L. O'Hara, PA-C, Physician Assistant, Hospital Internal Medicine, Mayo Clinic Arizona, Phoenix, Arizona

Jenna Rolfs, DMSc, PA-C, Program Director, University of Lynchburg School of PA Medicine, Lynchburg, Virginia

Daniel John Schreck, PA-C, Physician Assistant, Hospital Internal Medicine, Mayo Clinic Arizona, Phoenix, Arizona

Ashlyn Smith, PA-C, Endocrinology Associates, P.A., Scottsdale, Arizona; President, American Society of Endocrine Physician Assistants; Adjunct Assistant Professor, Physician Assistant Program, Midwestern University College of Health Sciences, Glendale, Arizona

Amanda Stark, PA-C, Physician Assistant, Hospital Internal Medicine, Mayo Clinic Arizona, Phoenix, Arizona

Kurt Tengberg, MS, PA-C, Adjunct Assistant Professor, Physician Assistant Program, Midwestern University College of Health Sciences, Glendale, Arizona

Amy K. Thompson, ARNP, AANP-C, International Volunteer Medical Provider, Coeur d'Alene, Idaho

Elyse Watkins, DHSc, PA-C, DFAAPA, Associate Professor, University of Lynchburg School of PA Medicine, Lynchburg, Virginia

Marion Weich, BA, BS, MEdA, PA-C, Physician Assistant, Scottsdale Gastroenterology Associates, Scottsdale, Arizona

Foreword

This year celebrates my 49th year in the physician assistant (PA) profession and my 26th year in PA education. I look back at the origins of the profession (circa 1965) when Dr. Eugene Stead, Jr., Dr. Richard Smith, and other pioneers sought to solve a lack and maldistribution of healthcare providers in this country, and I am still struck by their forward thinking. They created opportunities for highly skilled military medics and corpsmen, which would become the foundation of the PA profession. In those early decades, individuals with a great deal of passion and dedication created, advanced, and led our professional organizations on both state and national levels and even international level. The attainment of licensure and authority were the highlights of these early years. Now that the profession is recognized for its essential role in the U.S. healthcare system and our contributions to quality, accessible, and affordable patient care, it is time to ensure that the standards for our profession remain high.

This leads me to the authors of this important book. Eve Hoover, Kimberly Carter, Robyn Sears, and Sarah Bolander are talented and tested PA educators with a combined 55 years in clinical practice and decades in medical education. They understand that the first door to open to a career as a PA is certification and that preparation can involve long, grueling hours of review. However, the authors would like to flip that perspective and suggest that preparation need not be brutal but fun. Having spent years preparing students for national and regional Challenge Bowls, they took their expertise and channeled it into a Challenge Bowl–style review of quick-answer questions designed to supplement exam preparations during PA school and through preparation for PANCE/PANRE. This book is designed not as a sit-down-and-read text but rather one to carry with you to use during those small sessions of downtime in your schedule. It is also a great resource for group studying. This is a real-world practical book that will test and increase your knowledge in all the areas of medicine important to your practice.

Becoming competent in medicine requires cognitive, integrative, relational, and affective/moral skills. Remaining competent is certainly developmental in the context of lifelong learning. This book provides foundational knowledge to assist in each of those competency areas. Learning is neither static nor a sprint but rather a marathon throughout one's career. Mastery or expertise is achieved by the continuous acquisition of knowledge coupled with sound practice and experience.

Once again, this book will be an invaluable asset to a PA student or the brand-new PA and the seasoned professional who seeks to gain insight and lifelong learning in their practice. I continue to be proud of our profession and the pioneers leading us into new frontiers.

Onward and upward!

Randy D. Danielsen, PhD, PA-C Emeritus, DFAAPA
Professor and Director, Doctor of Medical Science Program
Arizona School of Health Science
Director, The Center for the Future of the Health Professions
A.T. Still University, Mesa, Arizona

Preface

Passion for the PA profession and a love for teaching and learning pedagogies sparked our development of *PANCE/PANRE Challenge: Quick Q&A Review*. We are PAs and educators who enthusiastically support the advancement of the PA profession on the state and national levels, and proactively seek opportunities to assist learners in the development of critical thinking skills and clinical acumen. We have a combined 55 years of varied clinical experience in the fields of family medicine, college health, internal medicine, gastroenterology and nutrition, emergency medicine, pain management, orthopaedics, dermatology, and oncology. We strive to bring relevancy, clarity, and enhanced learning opportunities by interweaving didactic knowledge with pearls related to clinical practice. Additionally, we have spent years on state and national PA continuing medical education committees and are nationally recognized speakers on various clinical and educational topics. We are University Challenge Bowl faculty advisors for state and national competitions and routinely engage in exam question writing in our role as PA educators. This book was inspired by hundreds of PA students that we are honored to coach during challenge bowl practice. The students are always enthusiastic and eager to learn through an interactive Q&A format.

PANCE/PANRE Challenge: Quick Q&A Review is a comprehensive book of quick-answer questions designed to supplement exam preparation at various stages from the didactic year through to the PANCE and PANRE exams. Through educating and mentoring hundreds of students, it became apparent to us that learners can never have enough opportunities to answer practice questions. *PANCE/PANRE Challenge: Quick Q&A Review* includes 1,000 questions to bring learners' awareness to their strengths, discover gaps in understanding, and encourage self-directed learning. This resource was intentionally designed without use of distractors to encourage the learner to think quickly without prompting, as expected in clinical practice. This up to date, evidence-based, user-friendly resource will benefit PA students in training and preparing for the PANCE, clinicians staying abreast of medical knowledge and with PANRE preparation, and PA educators searching to expand strategies for student support. This book can also serve as a resource for students preparing for the didactic and clinical year assessments, OSCEs, and rotation exams.

Learners can self-reflect, recognizing areas of strength and concepts that may require further exploration with supplemental materials. We strategically incorporated a combination of recall questions along with higher-order questions that require the learner to apply and analyze clinical information. For higher-order questions, brief explanations for the correct answer are provided to describe concepts and encourage the learner to initiate further self-directed exploration to solidify concepts. The supplemental, innovative online resource, ExamPrepConnect, provides learners with an additional method to practice assessment on the go and motivates the learner with an interactive flashcard feature.

We enjoyed the opportunity to develop this resource, working with so many talented PA colleagues in a variety of specialties. As the PA profession has recently been named the #1 U.S. Best Job by *U.S. News and World Report*, our enthusiasm for our great profession grows, and the need for additional evidence-based, user-friendly, relevant educational resources continues. Thank you for selecting this book and for all the work you do making our profession #1. Good luck in your current and future professional endeavors.

All our best,
Eve B. Hoover, DMSc, PA-C, DFAAPA
Kimberly A. Carter, DMSc, PA-C, RD
Robyn A. Sears, DMSc, PA-C
Sarah L. Bolander, DMSc, PA-C, DFAAPA

Pass Guarantee

If you use this resource to prepare for your exam and you do not pass, you may return it for a refund of your full purchase price. To receive a refund, you must return your product along with a copy of your original receipt and exam score report. Product must be returned and received within 180 days of the original purchase date. Excludes tax, shipping, and handling. One offer per person and address. Refunds will be issued within eight weeks from acceptance and approval. This offer is valid for US residents only. Void where prohibited. To begin the process, please contact customer service at CS@springerpub.com.

Introduction

▶ PANCE/PANRE

The Physician Assistant National Certifying Exam (PANCE) is the initial certification exam developed by the National Commission on Certification of Physician Assistants (NCCPA). This exam includes 300 multiple-choice questions, and the test-taker is given 5 hours to complete the exam. The Physician Assistant National Recertification Exam (PANRE) is taken by certified PAs who have previously passed the PANCE to maintain certification. The timing of this exam is during the 9th or 10th year of the recertification cycle. The PANRE format varies from the PANCE in number of questions and timing.

Both the PANCE and PANRE include questions related to each organ system and are delineated by Task Areas as outlined in Table I.1. The specific conditions and categories covered in the PANCE and PANRE are outlined in the 2019 NCCPA Content Blueprint.

▶ HOW TO USE THIS BOOK

PANCE/PANRE Q&A Challenge: Quick Q&A Review is organized according to the NCCPA Content Blueprint by organ system. The quantity of questions in each organ system and within each task area are weighted based on the blueprint percentages. Table I.1 summarizes the breakdown of content. This allows the learner to pinpoint both organ systems and task areas that require further self-directed exploration. This resource also includes a variety of cognitive difficulty increasing from recall questions to higher-order questions (apply and analyze). The recall questions do not include an explanation since these are first-order concepts. The apply and analyze questions require the reader to utilize clinical reasoning and clinical judgment skills to answer the question. A brief explanation is then provided to guide the learner and support further knowledge acquisition.

This book is organized by body system as outlined by the NCCPA Content Blueprint. Furthermore, each question identifies the task area addressed, with the exception of the professional practice questions. To simplify studying, professional practice is a stand-alone chapter that encompasses 5% of this book.

The questions in this book are designed as bound flashcards, in which questions are on the front page and answers are on the flip page directly opposite their related questions. This allows for quick access to the answers and immediate remediation. The questions are Challenge Bowl style, which means answers are short, quick, and direct. The book can be used for individual study, or in groups for team-based, game-style learning.

▶ **ExamPrepConnect**

Purchase of the print product provides 6-month access to Springer Publishing's ExamPrepConnect interactive digital exam preparation platform. You will find there all of the questions in this book available to you in digital flashcard format for study on the go. Details for how to access ExamPrepConnect appear on the tear-out card at the front of this book.

▶ **CONCLUSION**

PANCE/PANRE Q&A Challenge: Quick Q&A Review was inspired and designed to allow students and clinicians to self-reflect on areas of expertise and recognize gaps in knowledge to encourage learners to proactively seek opportunities for continuing education and professional development.

Table I.1 Question Breakdown by NCCPA Content Blueprint Task and Organ System

Task / Organ Systems	History Taking and Performing Physical Examination 17%	Using Diagnostic and Laboratory Studies 12%	Formulating Most Likely Diagnosis 18%	Health Maintenance, Patient Education, and Preventive Measures 10%	Clinical Intervention 14%	Pharmaceutical Therapeutics 14%	Applying Basic Scientific Concepts 10%	Professional Practice 5%	% of Exam	# of Qs
Cardiovascular System	22	16	23	13	18	18	13		13%	123
Dermatologic System	9	6	9	5	7	7	5		5%	48
Endocrine System	12	8	12	7	10	10	7		7%	66
Eyes, Ears, Nose, and Throat	12	8	12	7	10	10	7		7%	66
Gastrointestinal System/Nutrition	15	11	16	9	13	13	9		9%	86
Genitourinary System (Male and Female)	9	6	9	5	7	7	5		5%	48
Hematologic System	9	6	9	5	7	7	5		5%	48
Infectious Diseases	10	8	11	7	8	8	6		6%	58
Musculoskeletal System	14	10	14	8	11	11	8		8%	76
Neurologic System	12	8	12	7	10	10	7		7%	66
Psychiatry/Behavioral Science	10	8	11	7	8	8	6		6%	58
Pulmonary System	17	12	18	10	14	14	10		10%	95
Renal System	9	6	9	5	7	7	5		5%	48
Reproductive System (Male and Female)	12	8	12	7	10	10	7		7%	66
								48		48
TOTAL	172	120	179	101	140	140	100	48	100%	1000

Cardiovascular System

1. A 28-year-old man presents to the emergency department with low-grade fever, mild dyspnea, and anterior pleuritic chest pain that is relieved by leaning forward. He recently had a self-limited viral upper respiratory infection. What is the classic cardiac auscultation finding associated with the presumptive diagnosis?

2. What is the most dangerous bleeding complication associated with use of thrombolytic medications?

3. A 73-year-old man with hypertension and kidney dysfunction, treated with angiotensin-converting enzyme (ACE) inhibitor, is found to have peaked T waves on electrocardiogram (ECG). What is the most likely electrolyte disturbance causing this ECG abnormality?

4. In a patient with recurrent ventricular tachycardia who has a typical outflow tract on electrocardiogram and normal heart structure, besides beta-blockers, what other class of medication is recommended as suppressive therapy?

5. What is the most common cause of restrictive cardiomyopathy?

6. What class of medication should be avoided in treatment of acute decompensated heart failure due to its immediate negative ionotropic effects?

7. A healthy post-menopausal 56-year-old woman presents to the emergency department with chest pain, pressure, and shortness of breath 2 days after unexpectedly losing her husband. Her electrocardiogram reveals ST-segment elevation in anterior precordial leads and T-wave inversion. The chest radiograph is normal. Initial cardiac enzymes are abnormal, and cardiac catheterization shows no coronary artery abnormality. What other finding on cardiac catheterization would confirm the presumptive diagnosis?

8. What is the heart's normal pacemaker located in the right atrium?

9. A 13-year-old girl with tall stature, wide arm span, and scoliosis presents to the clinic for a follow-up visit of her chronic condition. Family members have similar physical features and have been found to have mutations in the fibrillin gene (*FBN1*) on chromosome 15. What is the primary indication for an echocardiogram obtained at least annually?

1. Pericardial friction rub
The clinical vignette supports the diagnosis of acute pericarditis. The most common cause is a viral infection leading to inflammation of the pericardial tissue.
Blueprint Task: *History Taking and Performing Physical Examination*
Cognitive Level: *Analyze*

2. Intracranial bleeding
Blueprint Task: *Pharmaceutical Therapeutics*
Cognitive Level: *Recall*

3. Hyperkalemia
While peaked T waves are a common finding in patients with hyperkalemia, electrocardiogram (ECG) may also be completely normal.
Blueprint Task: *Formulating Most Likely Diagnosis*
Cognitive Level: *Apply*

4. Nondihydropyridine calcium channel blockers
Beta-blockers and nondihydropyridine calcium channel blockers are typically used as suppressive medications. If suppressive medications are not effective in preventing recurrence, catheter ablation is recommended.
Blueprint Task: *Clinical Intervention*
Cognitive Level: *Apply*

5. Amyloidosis
Blueprint Task: *Applying Basic Scientific Concepts*
Cognitive Level: *Recall*

6. Beta-blockers
Blueprint Task: *Pharmaceutical Therapeutics*
Cognitive Level: *Recall*

7. Left ventricular apical ballooning
The clinical vignette supports the diagnosis of stress cardiomyopathy (Takotsubo syndrome), which classically follows severe emotional or physical stress.
Blueprint Task: *Using Diagnostic and Laboratory Studies*
Cognitive Level: *Analyze*

8. Sinoatrial (SA) node
Blueprint Task: *Applying Basic Scientific Concepts*
Cognitive Level: *Recall*

9. Monitor aortic root diameter
The clinical vignette supports the diagnosis of Marfan syndrome. Risk of aortic root dilation predisposes patients to dissection.
Blueprint Task: *Health Maintenance, Patient Education, and Preventive Measures*
Cognitive Level: *Analyze*

10. A 29-year-old man with a history of injection drug use presents to the emergency department with fever, chills, and dyspnea. Echocardiogram reveals vegetation on the tricuspid valve. What are the hemorrhagic nontender lesions that may be present on the palms or soles in this patient?

11. Besides fibrates, what other lipid-lowering medication is indicated for the treatment of severe hypertriglyceridemia?

12. What is the most common cause of congestive heart failure (CHF)?

13. An asymptomatic 55-year-old patient comes in for an annual physical. Electrocardiogram (ECG) reveals a PR interval of >200 ms but is otherwise normal. What is the recommended treatment for this condition?

14. What diagnosis is defined by chronic lung disease with pulmonary hypertension leading to right ventricular cardiac dysfunction?

15. A healthy 22-year-old woman with scoliosis presents to the clinic with occasional chest pain and palpitations. Cardiac auscultation reveals a mid-systolic click. What study will confirm the presumptive diagnosis?

16. What form of dyspnea is characterized by exacerbation in the recumbent position and improves with elevation of the upper body?

17. What is the most common congenital heart defect diagnosed in infancy?

18. At which anatomic location of the chest are pulmonic heart sounds best auscultated?

(See answers next page.)

10. Janeway lesions

The clinical vignette supports the diagnosis of infective endocarditis. In addition to Janeway lesions, other cutaneous findings may include Osler's nodes (painful nodules on fingers) and splinter hemorrhages.
Blueprint Task: History Taking and Performing Physical Examination
Cognitive Level: Apply

11. Omega-3 fatty acids

Blueprint Task: Pharmaceutical Therapeutics
Cognitive Level: Recall

12. Ischemic heart disease

Blueprint Task: Applying Basic Scientific Concepts
Cognitive Level: Recall

13. No specific therapy indicated

The ECG findings are consistent with a first-degree atrioventricular block, which does not require therapy in asymptomatic patients.
Blueprint Task: Clinical Intervention
Cognitive Level: Apply

14. Cor pulmonale

Blueprint Task: Formulating Most Likely Diagnosis
Cognitive Level: Recall

15. Echocardiogram

The clinical vignette supports the diagnosis of mitral valve prolapse (MVP). MVP is often suspected by history and physical exam alone; however, many patients may be asymptomatic.
Blueprint Task: Using Diagnostic and Laboratory Studies
Cognitive Level: Apply

16. Orthopnea

Blueprint Task: History Taking and Performing Physical Examination
Cognitive Level: Recall

17. Ventricular septal defect (VSD)

VSD is an acyanotic heart defect, resulting in pulmonary hypertension and congestion. VSD presents as a holosystolic murmur at the lower left sternal border. Bicuspid aortic valve is considered the most common congenital heart defect; however, it may not alter hemodynamics and remains undetected until later in life.
Blueprint Task: Applying Basic Scientific Concepts
Cognitive Level: Apply

18. Left second intercostal space at the sternal border

Blueprint Task: History Taking and Performing Physical Examination
Cognitive Level: Recall

19. A 68-year-old man develops pleuritic chest pain 5 days after sustaining a myocardial infarction. Chest discomfort improves with leaning forward. Assuming his symptoms are caused by an inflammatory reaction of the pericardium, what two medications are recommended for the presumptive diagnosis?

20. A 39-year-old woman has premature ventricular contractions (PVCs) but is asymptomatic without associated cardiac disease. What is the best patient education regarding the management of this condition?

21. What is the primary imaging study recommended for initial abdominal aortic aneurysm screening?

22. What is a rare neuroendocrine tumor, similar to a pheochromocytoma, that may present with chest pain if located in the mediastinum but is more commonly localized to the head or neck?

23. What class of lipid-lowering medication can interfere with the absorption of fat-soluble vitamins?

24. A 22-year-old patient presents to the clinic with intractable vomiting and diarrhea. Vital signs reveal a blood pressure of 120/80 mm Hg supine with a heart rate of 80 bpm. Within 3 minutes of standing, the blood pressure drops to 95/70 mm Hg and heart rate increases to 100 bpm. What term describes these vital sign changes?

25. In the management of superficial thrombophlebitis, in addition to heat and elevation, what class of medication is recommended?

26. A patient presents to the emergency department with a suspected ruptured abdominal aortic aneurysm. Fluid resuscitation is started to maintain sufficient organ perfusion. What approach to blood pressure management may minimize hemorrhage?

27. What is the most common cause of cardiogenic shock?

(See answers next page.)

19. Aspirin and colchicine

The clinical vignette supports the diagnosis of Dressler's syndrome, which is a pericarditis following cardiac injury.
Blueprint Task: Pharmaceutical Therapeutics
Cognitive Level: Apply

20. Reassurance

Pharmacologic therapy is not indicated in asymptomatic patients. Beta-blockers or calcium channel blockers may be used in patients with symptomatic PVCs.
Blueprint Task: Health Maintenance, Patient Education, and Preventive Measures
Cognitive Level: Apply

21.Ultrasound

Blueprint Task: Clinical Intervention
Cognitive Level: Recall

22. Paraganglioma

Symptomatic patients with paraganglioma often experience hypertension, headache, palpitations, and diaphoresis. Paraganglioma has a strong potential for metastasis.
Blueprint Task: Formulating Most Likely Diagnosis
Cognitive Level: Apply

23. Bile acid binding resins

Blueprint Task: Pharmaceutical Therapeutics
Cognitive Level: Recall

24. Orthostatic hypotension

Orthostatic hypotension, common in dehydration, is defined as a drop of systolic BP by ≥ 20 mm Hg or a decrease in diastolic BP of ≥ 10 mm Hg.
Blueprint Task: History Taking and Performing Physical Examination
Cognitive Level: Apply

25. Nonsteroidal anti-inflammatory drugs (NSAIDs)

Blueprint Task: Pharmaceutical Therapeutics
Cognitive Level: Recall

26. Permissive hypotension

Management of ruptured abdominal aortic aneurysm requires a balance of fluid resuscitation and permissive hypotension to mitigate worsening hemorrhage.
Blueprint Task: Clinical Intervention
Cognitive Level: Apply

27. Myocardial infarction

Blueprint Task: Applying Basic Scientific Concepts
Cognitive Level: Recall

28. What is the interpretation of the following electrocardiogram (ECG) and is a pathogno-monic finding in patients with a pericardial effusion?

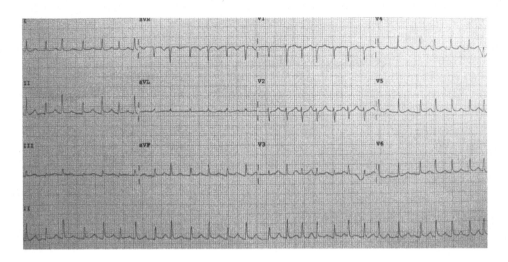

29. Following placement of an implantable cardioverter defibrillator (ICD) for recurring ventricular tachycardia, what mental health issue should be monitored in patients requiring repeated shocks?

30. What is the initial pharmacologic class of medication recommended for patients with symptomatic tricuspid stenosis?

31. A 19-year-old basketball player is urgently evaluated for chest pain, dyspnea, and syn-cope that developed during a strenuous practice. An echocardiogram reveals increased thickness of the left ventricular wall. What is the presumptive diagnosis?

32. What therapy can be worn daily to prevent and reduce lower extremity edema associ-ated with chronic venous insufficiency?

33. What is the preferred cardiac biomarker used in the diagnosis of acute myocardial infarction (MI) due to its sensitivity, specificity, and detectability?

34. A newborn is delivered at 30 weeks gestation. Cardiac exam reveals a continuous machine-like murmur and precordial thrill. What is the first-line pharmacologic ther-apy for the presumptive diagnosis?

35. What is the expected ejection fraction in a patient with heart failure with preserved ejection fraction (HFpEF)?

36. A patient was recently discharged from the hospital following admission for acute dehydration requiring intravenous (IV) fluid replacement. He now has an erythema-tous, tender induration along a superficial vein in his forearm. What clinical condition is represented by this physical exam finding?

(See answers next page.)

28. Electrical alternans

Electrical alternans results from the heart swaying within the effusion.
Blueprint Task: Using Diagnostic and Laboratory Studies
Cognitive Level: Apply

29. Post-traumatic stress disorder (PTSD)

Repeated shocks from an ICD, even if appropriate, may result in PTSD.
Blueprint Task: Health Maintenance, Patient Education, and Preventive Measures
Cognitive Level: Apply

30. Diuretics

Blueprint Task: Pharmaceutical Therapeutics
Cognitive Level: Recall

31. Hypertrophic cardiomyopathy

Hypertrophic cardiomyopathy is characterized by left ventricular wall thickness and associated sequelae, increasing risk of sudden death.
Blueprint Task: Formulating Most Likely Diagnosis
Cognitive Level: Apply

32. Compression stockings

Blueprint Task: Clinical Intervention
Cognitive Level: Recall

33. High-sensitivity troponin testing

Troponin I and T are released during an acute MI. Troponin is detectable within hours after the onset. Troponin levels should continue to be monitored as the patient's condition evolves.
Blueprint Task: Using Diagnostic and Laboratory Studies
Cognitive Level: Apply

34. Indomethacin

The clinical vignette supports the diagnosis of patent ductus arteriosus (PDA). Indomethacin blocks the production of prostaglandins, ostensibly causing closure of the ductus arteriosus. If patency persists after indomethacin, surgical intervention may be required.
Blueprint Task: Pharmaceutical Therapeutics
Cognitive Level: Analyze

35. >50%

Blueprint Task: Applying Basic Scientific Concepts
Cognitive Level: Recall

36. Superficial thrombophlebitis

Localized tenderness, erythema, and swelling in an extremity following recent IV placement are indicative of superficial thrombophlebitis.
Blueprint Task: History Taking and Performing Physical Examination
Cognitive Level: Apply

37. A 21-year-old woman presents to the clinic for phlebotomy. She develops sweating and lightheadedness followed by syncope. What type of syncope does this represent?

38. A 33-year-old woman presents to the clinic with increasing palpitations. The episodes now occur daily for brief periods. She denies any other symptoms and has a normal laboratory workup. The electrocardiogram in the office is negative for arrhythmia. What is the next best step to detect the underlying cause of her symptom?

39. What is the leading cause of mitral stenosis?

40. A 62-year-old man with a BMI of 32 kg/m² and a history of deep vein thrombosis (DVT) 2 years ago presents to the clinic with chronic swelling, itching, and discoloration of the legs. Physical exam reveals lower-extremity 1+ pitting edema and brawny hyperpigmentation without varicosities. The distal pulses are 2+ and equal. What is the presumptive diagnosis?

41. What is the primary reperfusion therapy for patients with ST-elevation myocardial infarction (STEMI)?

42. A 68-year-old woman is admitted to the hospital with stress cardiomyopathy. Besides aspirin and an angiotensin-converting enzyme (ACE) inhibitor, what other class of medication is recommended in the early treatment of this condition?

43. What biochemical marker should be measured during a workup of a patient who has suffered blunt chest wall trauma?

44. In addition to good oral hygiene, what education is necessary to discuss prior to a dental procedure for patients with a prosthetic heart valve?

45. What class of medication is the mainstay of treatment for congenital long QT syndrome to reduce the risk of sudden cardiac death?

(See answers next page.)

37. Vasovagal
Blueprint Task: Formulating Most Likely Diagnosis
Cognitive Level: Recall

38. Ambulatory electrocardiogram (ECG) monitoring device
Ambulatory devices allow for outpatient monitoring of palpitations over an extended period. Monitors may be wearable, handheld, or patch.
Blueprint Task: Clinical Intervention
Cognitive Level: Apply

39. Rheumatic fever
Blueprint Task: Applying Basic Scientific Concepts
Cognitive Level: Recall

40. Chronic venous insufficiency
Prior history of DVT, leg injury, and obesity increase the likelihood of developing chronic venous insufficiency.
Blueprint Task: Formulating Most Likely Diagnosis
Cognitive Level: Apply

41. Percutaneous coronary intervention (PCI)
Blueprint Task: Clinical Intervention
Cognitive Level: Recall

42. Beta-blocker
Patients with stress (also known as Takotsubo) cardiomyopathy are typically treated with aspirin, beta-blockers, and ACE inhibitors or angiotensin II receptor blockers (ARBs) until left ventricular function fully recovers.
Blueprint Task: Pharmaceutical Therapeutics
Cognitive Level: Apply

43. Troponin I
Blueprint Task: Clinical Intervention
Cognitive Level: Recall

44. Antibiotic prophylaxis
Antibiotic prophylaxis is required in high-risk patients for endocarditis prevention.
Blueprint Task: Health Maintenance, Patient Education, and Preventive Measures
Cognitive Level: Apply

45. Beta-blockers
Blueprint Task: Clinical Intervention
Cognitive Level: Recall

46. A 33-year-old man is taken to the emergency department with chest pain and dyspnea following a motor vehicle accident. Physical exam reveals hypotension and bruising of the chest, muffled heart sounds, and jugular venous distension (JVD). What is the initial cardiac imaging study recommended in this patient to evaluate for the presumptive diagnosis?

47. What is the most common arrhythmia leading to sudden cardiac death?

48. A 49-year-old man with a 40-pack-year tobacco history presents to the emergency department with 2 days of progressive pain and swelling of the left lower leg since returning to the United States from China. There is no history of trauma, chest pain, or shortness of breath. Vital signs are stable. What is the preferred diagnostic study to evaluate for the presumptive diagnosis?

49. What class of medication is recommended to avoid in patients with a history of cocaine use experiencing acute coronary syndrome (ACS)?

50. What is a potential side effect of abrupt discontinuation of clonidine in a patient who has been taking it for several years?

51. A 79-year-old man with peripheral vascular disease, claudication, and tobacco use presents to the emergency department with a sudden onset of left lower extremity pain and numbness. Physical exam reveals left lower extremity pallor, coolness, and absent distal pulses. What is the most likely diagnosis?

52. Which leads on an electrocardiogram represent the inferior wall of the heart?

53. What is the minimum amount of time a patient who has recently undergone percutaneous coronary intervention (PCI) with placement of a bare metal stent should be kept on dual anti-platelet therapy (DAPT)?

54. What pulse is palpated on the medial side of the dorsum of the foot?

(See answers next page.)

46. Extended focused assessment with sonography for trauma (eFAST)

The clinical vignette supports the diagnosis of cardiac tamponade represented by Beck's triad (hypotension, muffled heart sounds, and JVD). In unstable patients, particularly those who have experienced trauma, the initial cardiac imaging recommended is an eFAST to assess for a pericardial effusion. In nontraumatic cardiac tamponade, echocardiography is recommended to confirm the diagnosis.

Blueprint Task: *Using Diagnostic and Laboratory Studies*
Cognitive Level: *Analyze*

47. Ventricular fibrillation

Blueprint Task: *Applying Basic Scientific Concepts*
Cognitive Level: *Recall*

48. Lower-extremity venous doppler ultrasound

The clinical vignette supports the diagnosis of deep vein thrombosis (DVT).

Blueprint Task: *Using Diagnostic and Laboratory Studies*
Cognitive Level: *Apply*

49. Beta-blockers

Beta-blockers have the potential to worsen coronary vasoconstriction.

Blueprint Task: *Clinical Intervention*
Cognitive Level: *Apply*

50. Rebound hypertension

Blueprint Task: *Pharmaceutical Therapeutics*
Cognitive Level: *Recall*

51. Acute arterial occlusion

The clinical vignette supports the diagnosis of acute arterial occlusion leading to ischemia. Immediate revascularization is required in symptomatic patients.

Blueprint Task: *Formulating Most Likely Diagnosis*
Cognitive Level: *Apply*

52. II, III, and aVF

Blueprint Task: *Using Diagnostic and Laboratory Studies*
Cognitive Level: *Recall*

53. 4 weeks

Patients who have undergone PCI with angioplasty should remain on DAPT for 2–4 weeks. Patients with a drug-eluting stent should remain on DAPT for at least 6 months to one year.

Blueprint Task: *Pharmaceutical Therapeutics*
Cognitive Level: *Apply*

54. Dorsalis pedis

Blueprint Task: *History Taking and Performing Physical Examination*
Cognitive Level: *Recall*

55. A patient with metastatic breast cancer is diagnosed with a proximal deep vein thrombosis (DVT) of the lower extremity. How long should anticoagulation therapy be recommended?

56. Which specialized test evaluates for ulnar artery patency prior to obtaining vascular access of the radial artery?

57. A 67-year-old man presents to the clinic with palpitations. The pulse is irregularly irregular. What test will confirm the presumptive disorder?

58. A patient with congestive heart failure is placed on furosemide to improve dyspnea and peripheral edema. What electrolyte must be monitored and supplemented as appropriate?

59. A man with ischemic chest pain firmly places a clenched fist over his sternum. What is the name of this sign?

60. A congenital bicuspid aortic valve increases the risk of developing what condition?

61. A 72-year-old man with acute coronary syndrome and severe left ventricular dysfunction has hypotension and decreased perfusion. What is the presumptive diagnosis?

62. What medication is contraindicated in patients with right ventricular, inferior wall myocardial infarction?

63. Why should a clinician avoid palpating both carotid pulses simultaneously?

(See answers next page.)

55. Indefinitely
There is a significant risk of recurrence of thrombus formation in patients with underlying malignancy.
Blueprint Task: Health Maintenance, Patient Education, and Preventive Measures
Cognitive Level: Apply

56. Allen test
Blueprint Task: History Taking and Performing Physical Examination
Cognitive Level: Recall

57. Electrocardiogram
The clinical vignette supports the diagnosis of atrial fibrillation. A serious consequence of atrial fibrillation includes thrombus formation and potential embolization.
Blueprint Task: Using Diagnostic and Laboratory Studies
Cognitive Level: Apply

58. Potassium
Loop diuretics are commonly used to reduce volume overload in patients with congestive heart failure. Following administration, renal function and hypokalemia should be monitored.
Blueprint Task: Clinical Intervention
Cognitive Level: Apply

59. Levine sign
Blueprint Task: History Taking and Performing Physical Examination
Cognitive Level: Recall

60. Aortic stenosis
The aortic valve is normally a tricuspid valve.
Blueprint Task: Applying Basic Scientific Concepts
Cognitive Level: Apply

61. Cardiogenic shock
Cardiogenic shock, caused by reduced cardiac output, is a leading cause of death in patients with acute myocardial infarction.
Blueprint Task: Formulating Most Likely Diagnosis
Cognitive Level: Apply

62. Nitroglycerin
Shock is a sequela of right ventricular infarction. Nitroglycerin reduces preload and may lead to hemodynamic instability.
Blueprint Task: Pharmaceutical Therapeutics
Cognitive Level: Apply

63. Risk of syncope
Blueprint Task: History Taking and Performing Physical Examination
Cognitive Level: Recall

64. What arrhythmia is demonstrated on the following electrocardiogram (ECG)?

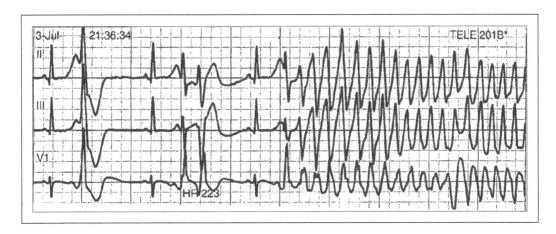

65. A 32-year-old woman presents to the clinic with progressive aching and heaviness in her legs since delivering her second child. Standing all day as a hairdresser increases symptoms. Physical exam of the lower extremities reveals dilated tortuous superficial vessels. In addition to leg elevation, what nonsurgical measure is recommended for symptom control?

66. Besides infection and tissue necrosis, what other common potential side effect might be expected in patients undergoing varicose vein sclerotherapy?

67. A 67-year-old man with poorly controlled hypertension and coronary artery disease presents to the emergency department with a 1-week history of worsening dyspnea, lower extremity swelling, and a 10-pound weight gain. He sleeps with more pillows and wakes up gasping for air. Physical exam reveals an S3 gallop, pulmonary rales, jugular vein distension, and 3+ pitting edema. What is the most likely diagnosis?

68. What is the most likely location for a stasis ulcer to develop in patients with chronic venous insufficiency and stasis dermatitis?

69. What procedure is typically indicated for symptomatic treatment of sinus node dysfunction?

70. A 62-year-old man with hypertension and tobacco use presents to the emergency department with sudden onset of severe, constant tearing anterior chest pain radiating to the back. On physical exam, he is hypertensive, and pulses in the extremities are decreased. Chest radiograph reveals a widened mediastinum and electrocardiogram is without ischemic changes. What bedside diagnostic imaging modality is recommended in the evaluation of the presumptive diagnosis?

71. What term defines a drop in the systolic BP of >10 mm Hg with inspiration that may occur in patients with cardiac tamponade?

(See answers next page.)

64. Torsades de pointes

Torsades de pointes, a congenital or acquired polymorphic tachycardia, is associated with a prolonged QT interval, and typically appears as a twisting of the QRS complex.

Blueprint Task: Using Diagnostic and Laboratory Studies
Cognitive Level: Apply

65. Elastic graduated compression stockings

The clinical vignette supports the diagnosis of varicose veins.

Blueprint Task: Health Maintenance, Patient Education, and Preventive Measures
Cognitive Level: Apply

66. Phlebitis

Blueprint Task: Health Maintenance, Patient Education, and Preventive Measures
Cognitive Level: Recall

67. Congestive heart failure

The history and physical exam findings support volume overload secondary to congestive heart failure.

Blueprint Task: Formulating Most Likely Diagnosis
Cognitive Level: Apply

68. Medial ankle

Blueprint Task: Applying Basic Scientific Concepts
Cognitive Level: Recall

69. Permanent pacemaker implantation

Patients with asymptomatic sinus node dysfunction (also known as sick sinus syndrome) usually do not require treatment.

Blueprint Task: Clinical Intervention
Cognitive Level: Apply

70. Transesophageal echocardiogram (TEE)

The clinical vignette supports the diagnosis of aortic dissection. TEE may be accomplished emergently but requires sedation due to esophageal intubation. CT or MR angiography are also effective for confirming dissection. Imaging modality choice is largely dependent on patient stability.

Blueprint Task: Using Diagnostic and Laboratory Studies
Cognitive Level: Analyze

71. Pulsus paradoxus

Blueprint Task: History Taking and Performing Physical Examination
Cognitive Level: Recall

72. A 5-year-old girl with Turner syndrome presents to the clinic. Her parents report that she is struggling to keep up with her friends on the playground. Physical exam reveals elevated blood pressures in upper extremity compared to lower extremity with delayed and weakened femoral pulses compared to brachial pulses. She also has a systolic ejection murmur. What is the most likely diagnosis?

73. A 77-year-old man with familial hypercholesterolemia presents for follow-up after recent percutaneous coronary intervention. Recent lab work reveals an LDL of 155 mg/dL. He is currently taking a high-intensity statin along with ezetimibe. What class of injectable medication is recommended to further reduce this patient's LDL?

74. An 81-year-old woman presents to the clinic with fatigue, worsening shoulder and hip pain, and morning stiffness. Symptoms improved markedly after only 3 days of low-dose prednisone. This patient is at a higher risk of developing what condition that commonly presents with new onset of headaches, change in vision, and jaw claudication?

75. What clinical intervention is the primary therapy for symptomatic arrhythmias that do not improve with pharmacologic treatment?

76. A patient recently suffered an anterior wall ST-elevation myocardial infarction and presented with a suspected secondary left ventricular aneurysm. What electrocardiogram (ECG) finding would support the diagnosis in this patient?

77. What is the most common type of benign cardiac tumor in adults?

78. A newborn is found to have a ventricular septal defect, pulmonic stenosis, right ventricular hypertrophy, and an overriding aorta. What is the most likely diagnosis?

79. What clinical intervention can be performed in the emergency department to increase survival in patients with cardiac tamponade?

(See answers next page.)

72. Coarctation of the aorta

Coarctation of the aorta should be considered in all younger patients with hypertension. Coarctation of the aorta may be more common in males but is also associated with Turner syndrome. Symptoms may not present until systemic hypertension leads to left ventricular heart failure.

Blueprint Task: *Formulating Most Likely Diagnosis*
Cognitive Level: *Analyze*

73. Proprotein convertase subtilisin/kexin type 9 (PCSK9) inhibitor

PCSK9 inhibitors lower LDL cholesterol levels and are recommended as an adjunct therapy to statins or in patients who are statin-intolerant.

Blueprint Task: *Pharmaceutical Therapeutics*
Cognitive Level: *Apply*

74. Giant cell arteritis

The clinical vignette supports the diagnosis of polymyalgia rheumatica (PMR). Giant cell arteritis is also known as temporal arteritis.

Blueprint Task: *Health Maintenance, Patient Education, and Preventive Measures*
Cognitive Level: *Analyze*

75. Catheter ablation

Blueprint Task: *Clinical Intervention*
Cognitive Level: *Recall*

76. Persistent ST-segment elevation

Aneurysms following myocardial infarction can be recognized with prolonged ST-segment elevation on ECG for up to 1–2 months and confirmed by echocardiogram.

Blueprint Task: *Using Diagnostic and Laboratory Studies*
Cognitive Level: *Apply*

77. Myxoma

Blueprint Task: *Applying Basic Scientific Concepts*
Cognitive Level: *Recall*

78. Tetralogy of Fallot (ToF)

ToF is a cyanotic congenital heart condition caused by blood flow from the right atrium to the left ventricle. Bottlenecking created by the pulmonary artery stenosis causes the majority of blood to be pumped to the left ventricle via the VSD, ultimately bypassing the lungs and oxygenation.

Blueprint Task: *Formulating Most Likely Diagnosis*
Cognitive Level: *Apply*

79. Pericardiocentesis

Blueprint Task: *Clinical Intervention*
Cognitive Level: *Recall*

80. What historical feature, classic in congestive heart failure, is defined by acute episodes of severe shortness of breath that disrupts sleep?

81. A 62-year-old woman presents to the clinic with chest pain at rest and is found to have transient ST-segment elevation caused by localized vasospasm of the coronary arteries. What is the most likely diagnosis?

82. What renovascular disease can contribute to secondary hypertension?

83. What is the classic electrocardiogram (ECG) finding associated with acute pericarditis?

84. A 65-year-old man presents to the emergency department with chest pain and blood pressure of 230/115 mm Hg. Electrocardiogram (ECG) reveals an acute anteroseptal myocardial infarction (MI). In addition to nitroglycerin, what pharmacologic class of medication is recommended?

85. What is the target therapeutic INR range for warfarin therapy in patients with a mechanical heart valve to prevent thromboembolic complications?

86. What specialized test involves the clinician placing firm pressure on the right upper quadrant under the edge of the ribs and maintaining pressure for approximately 10 seconds while assessing for jugular venous distension?

87. What diagnostic study should be performed prior to cardioversion in a patient with new-onset atrial fibrillation that began more than 48 hours ago?

88. A 60-year-old man presents with newly diagnosed pulmonary hypertension. Physical exam reveals a continuous and harsh sounding murmur, heard most prominently in late systole during S2, over the left first and second interspaces of the sternal border. The patient has a low diastolic blood pressure with a wide pulse pressure. Electrocardiogram demonstrates left ventricular hypertrophy. What is the presumptive diagnosis?

89. What noninvasive screening test is used to evaluate for peripheral vascular disease by calculating the measurement of the highest systolic pressure in the ankles and dividing it by the highest systolic pressure in the arms?

(See answers next page.)

80. Paroxysmal nocturnal dyspnea (PND)
Blueprint Task: History Taking and Performing Physical Examination
Cognitive Level: Recall

81. Vasospastic angina
Vasospastic angina is also known as Prinzmetal's variant angina (PVA). The coronary artery spasm and ischemia in PVA may lead to acute MI, arrhythmia, or sudden death.
Blueprint Task: Formulating Most Likely Diagnosis
Cognitive Level: Apply

82. Renal artery stenosis
Blueprint Task: Applying Basic Scientific Concepts
Cognitive Level: Recall

83. Diffuse ST-segment elevation
Blueprint Task: Using Diagnostic and Laboratory Studies
Cognitive Level: Recall

84. Beta-blocker
The recommended pharmacologic management for hypertensive emergency in the setting of myocardial ischemia and acute MI includes either nitroglycerin with esmolol or labetalol, or the combination of nicardipine and esmolol.
Blueprint Task: Pharmaceutical Therapeutics
Cognitive Level: Analyze

85. 2.5 to 3.5
Blueprint Task: Health Maintenance, Patient Education, and Preventive Measures
Cognitive Level: Recall

86. Hepatojugular reflux
Blueprint Task: History Taking and Performing Physical Examination
Cognitive Level: Recall

87. Transesophageal echocardiogram (TEE)
A TEE provides evidence that the left atrium is free of thrombus prior to cardioversion.
Blueprint Task: Using Diagnostic and Laboratory Studies
Cognitive Level: Apply

88. Patent ductus arteriosus (PDA)
The clinical vignette supports the diagnosis of PDA in an adult patient. Patients are often asymptomatic until advanced age.
Blueprint Task: Formulating Most Likely Diagnosis
Cognitive Level: Apply

89. Ankle-brachial index (ABI)
Blueprint Task: Clinical Intervention
Cognitive Level: Recall

90. A healthy 45-year-old man presents to the emergency department following a syncopal episode. He is alert and oriented but has mild shortness of breath and lightheadedness. Electrocardiogram reveals a normal sinus rhythm with a heart rate of 43 bpm. A complete blood count and comprehensive metabolic panel are unremarkable. What medication is recommended in the treatment of this condition?

91. Upon auscultation of the carotid artery, the clinician hears a whooshing sound associated with turbulent flow. What is the name of this physical exam finding?

92. What commonly recommended diet has been shown to reduce blood pressure and encourages the consumption of fruits, vegetables, legumes, whole grains, and nuts with minimal intake of red meat and sugar-containing foods?

93. What syndrome is commonly associated with a slurred upstroke of the QRS complex on electrocardiogram (ECG), as seen in the following figure?

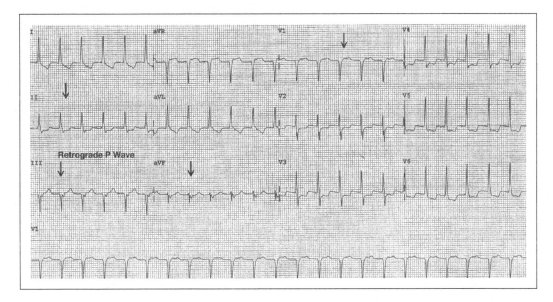

94. A 68-year-old man presents for evaluation following a syncopal episode. Cardiac exam reveals a palpable thrill and a loud systolic murmur, best heard at the left 2nd intercostal space radiating to the apex and neck. What valve is most likely affected?

95. What is the recommended age to begin assessing blood pressure in healthy children at well visits?

96. A 55-year-old man is admitted to the hospital with myositis along with moderately elevated creatine kinase levels. His current medications include carvedilol, aspirin, niacin, atorvastatin, and levothyroxine. Which combination of his medications is likely contributing to the diagnosis?

97. What is the pulse pressure in a patient with a blood pressure of 145/80 mm Hg?

(See answers next page.)

90. Atropine
The clinical vignette supports the diagnosis of symptomatic sinus bradycardia. Atropine aids in increasing heart rate.
Blueprint Task: Pharmaceutical Therapeutics
Cognitive Level: Apply

91. Bruit
Blueprint Task: History Taking and Performing Physical Examination
Cognitive Level: Recall

92. The Dietary Approaches to Stop Hypertension (DASH) diet
Blueprint Task: Health Maintenance, Patient Education, and Preventive Measures
Cognitive Level: Recall

93. Wolff–Parkinson–White Syndrome
The slurred upstroke of the QRS complex is called a delta wave.
Blueprint Task: Formulating Most Likely Diagnosis
Cognitive Level: Apply

94. Aortic
The clinical vignette supports the diagnosis of aortic valve stenosis.
Blueprint Task: History Taking and Performing Physical Examination
Cognitive Level: Apply

95. 3 years of age
Blueprint Task: Clinical Intervention
Cognitive Level: Recall

96. Atorvastatin and niacin
Muscle diseases such as myositis and rhabdomyolysis more commonly occur in patients on high-intensity statins taken along with certain drugs to include niacin, fibrates, erythromycin, antifungals, and cyclosporine.
Blueprint Task: Pharmaceutical Therapeutics
Cognitive Level: Apply

97. 65 mm Hg
Pulse pressure is measured by assessing the difference between systolic and diastolic pressures.
Blueprint Task: Applying Basic Scientific Concepts
Cognitive Level: Apply

98. What is the first-line class of medication that should be administered, following rapid defibrillation, to a patient in ventricular fibrillation?

99. A 50-year-old man develops fatigue and exertional dyspnea following a recent viral infection. Physical exam reveals tachycardia, hypotension, and fever. Electrocardiogram (ECG) reveals sinus tachycardia but is otherwise normal. Troponin is elevated. What is the most likely diagnosis?

100. What cardiac condition leads to a right-sided point of maximal impulse (PMI) due to abnormal position of the heart in the right chest cavity?

101. A 65-year-old woman has been receiving unfractionated heparin for the past 6 days. She presents today with a deep venous thrombosis in her distal lower extremity, bruising along the heparin injection site, and thrombocytopenia on her most recent lab work. What is the most likely cause of her symptoms?

102. An electrocardiogram (ECG) reveals a normal beat followed by a premature ventricular beat. If repeated, what is this pattern called?

103. A 69-year-old man with a history of chronic tobacco use presents for abdominal aortic aneurysm screening. What additional nonmodifiable factor places this patient at heightened risk for abdominal aortic aneurysm?

104. A 54-year-old man with hyperlipidemia and a 20-pack-year tobacco history presents to the emergency department with an episode of substernal chest pain while mowing the lawn that morning. He described the pain as a "tightness, squeezing, and burning." His pain lasted for 4 minutes and resolved with rest. He relates a history of similar episodes of chest pain with physical exertion. A follow-up electrocardiogram (ECG) is unremarkable. What is the most likely diagnosis?

105. A 76-year-old woman is admitted to the hospital with shortness of breath and pulmonary congestion. A diastolic murmur with an opening snap is present. Atrial and pulmonary capillary pressures are increased. Which heart valve is most likely affected in this patient?

106. What deviation from baseline, present in at least two adjacent leads, would be expected on electrocardiogram for the diagnosis of ST-elevation myocardial infarction (STEMI)?

(See answers next page.)

98. Vasopressors
Blueprint Task: *Clinical Intervention*
Cognitive Level: *Recall*

99. Myocarditis
Viral infection is a common cause of myocarditis. Myocarditis is typically a clinical diagnosis; however, an endomyocardial biopsy is the gold standard to confirm.
Blueprint Task: *Formulating Most Likely Diagnosis*
Cognitive Level: *Apply*

100. Dextrocardia
Blueprint Task: *History Taking and Performing Physical Examination*
Cognitive Level: *Recall*

101. Heparin-induced thrombocytopenia (HIT)
HIT occurs in patients most often 5–14 days after initial exposure, though it rarely can occur later. It is characterized by the presence of anti-heparin/PF4 antibodies, thrombocytopenia, localized skin changes, and potential thrombosis.
Blueprint Task: *Pharmaceutical Therapeutics*
Cognitive Level: *Apply*

102. Bigeminy
Blueprint Task: *Using Diagnostic and Laboratory Studies*
Cognitive Level: *Recall*

103. Family history
Blueprint Task: *Health Maintenance, Patient Education, and Preventive Measures*
Cognitive Level: *Recall*

104. Stable angina
The clinical vignette supports the diagnosis of stable angina, transient episodes of chest pain relieved with rest. The patient's history of hyperlipidemia and tobacco use raise the concern for atherosclerotic disease.
Blueprint Task: *Formulating Most Likely Diagnosis*
Cognitive Level: *Apply*

105. Mitral
The clinical vignette supports the diagnosis of mitral valve stenosis.
Blueprint Task: *History Taking and Performing Physical Examination*
Cognitive Level: *Apply*

106. >0.1 mV of ST elevation
Blueprint Task: *Using Diagnostic and Laboratory Studies*
Cognitive Level: *Recall*

107. A 72-year-old man is found to have a soft, high-pitched diastolic decrescendo murmur most clearly identified in the third intercostal space at the sternal border. A wide pulse pressure and a Corrigan pulse are present. What is the most likely valvular disorder causing these findings?

108. When comparing both the upper and lower extremity blood pressures (BP) in patients with coarctation of the aorta, what would be the expected finding?

109. What is the initial treatment goal for blood pressure reduction in patients with hypertensive emergency?

110. What is the expected timeframe for color to return to distal capillary beds following direct pressure causing blanching?

111. What chest radiograph finding is associated with a large thoracic aortic aneurysm?

112. A healthy 38-year-old woman presents to the emergency department with atraumatic chest pain. The pain is reproducible upon palpation of the anterior chest wall along the left sternal border at the second and third ribs. Cardiology workup is negative. What is the most likely diagnosis?

113. In addition to encouraging muscle-strengthening activities, what is the minimum number of minutes recommended to spend per week on moderate-intensity exercise?

114. What is the lowest grade murmur, accompanied by a palpable thrill, that can be diagnostically classified?

115. A 71-year-old man receives a heart transplant. What is the most likely cause of death within 3 years of this surgical procedure?

116. In patients who develop a cough after initiation of angiotensin-converting enzyme (ACE) inhibitor therapy, what class of medication is often recommended as a replacement?

(See answers next page.)

107. Chronic aortic regurgitation (AR)

A Corrigan pulse (also called water hammer pulse) is characterized by a forceful pulse followed by collapse.

Blueprint Task: Formulating Most Likely Diagnosis
Cognitive Level: Apply

108. Lower extremity BP < upper extremity BP

Blueprint Task: History Taking and Performing Physical Examination
Cognitive Level: Recall

109. Reduction of mean blood pressure by 25%

Blueprint Task: Clinical Intervention
Cognitive Level: Recall

110. < 2 seconds

The physical exam technique described assesses a normal capillary refill time (CRT)

Blueprint Task: History Taking and Performing Physical Examination
Cognitive Level: Apply

111. Widened mediastinum

Blueprint Task: Using Diagnostic and Laboratory Studies
Cognitive Level: Recall

112. Tietze syndrome

Tietze syndrome is caused by inflammation of the costochondral joints and is localized to the ribs that articulate at the sternum, most commonly involving the 2nd and 3rd ribs.

Blueprint Task: Formulating Most Likely Diagnosis
Cognitive Level: Apply

113. 150 minutes

Blueprint Task: Health Maintenance, Patient Education, and Preventive Measures
Cognitive Level: Recall

114. Grade 4

Gradation of murmurs is determined by sound intensity and existence of thrill.

Blueprint Task: History Taking and Performing Physical Examination
Cognitive Level: Apply

115. Graft rejection

Blueprint Task: Formulating Most Likely Diagnosis
Cognitive Level: Recall

116. Angiotensin II receptor blocker (ARB)

Blueprint Task: Health Maintenance, Patient Education, and Preventive Measures
Cognitive Level: Recall

117. A 30-year-old man presents with fever and acute migratory joint pain. The patient had a sore throat a month prior. Physical exam reveals a systolic murmur that is best heard at the 5th intercostal space at the left midclavicular line and radiates to the left axilla. Erythrocyte sedimentation rate (ESR) is elevated, and anti-streptolysin (ASO) antibodies are positive. What is the presumptive diagnosis?

118. What term defines elevated blood pressure with end-organ damage?

119. In patients with symptomatic peripheral artery disease affecting the lower extremities, what is the most commonly occurring manifestation?

120. Upon auscultation, what anatomic area of the chest will a murmur, secondary to tricuspid valve stenosis, be most prominent?

121. A 78-year-old man is brought to the emergency department via ambulance with an acute onset of severe abdominal pain. Physical exam reveals hypotension and a pulsatile abdominal mass. What is the presumptive diagnosis?

122. What syndrome increases the risk for adverse cardiovascular outcomes and is defined by abdominal obesity, hypertension, dyslipidemia, and insulin resistance?

123. What two pharmacologic classes of medication are recommended in the treatment of dilated cardiomyopathy?

(See answers next page.)

117. Acute rheumatic fever

An autoimmune reaction to prior infection with group A streptococcus can lead to acute rheumatic fever (ARF), which can manifest across multiple systems, including cardiac.
Blueprint Task: Formulating Most Likely Diagnosis
Cognitive Level: Apply

118. Hypertensive emergency

Blueprint Task: Formulating Most Likely Diagnosis
Cognitive Level: Recall

119. Intermittent claudication

Blueprint Task: History Taking and Performing Physical Examination
Cognitive Level: Recall

120. Left, lower sternal border

Blueprint Task: History Taking and Performing Physical Examination
Cognitive Level: Recall

121. Ruptured abdominal aortic aneurysm (AAA)

Classic triad of symptoms for a ruptured AAA includes hypotension, pulsatile abdominal mass, and abdominal or flank pain. Clinical suspicion for AAA must be identified early with any of these symptoms due to the rapid progression and life-threatening risk.
Blueprint Task: Formulating Most Likely Diagnosis
Cognitive Level: Apply

122. Metabolic syndrome

Blueprint Task: Formulating Most Likely Diagnosis
Cognitive Level: Recall

123. Beta-blockers and angiotensin-converting enzyme (ACE) inhibitors

Blueprint Task: Pharmaceutical Therapeutics
Cognitive Level: Recall

Dermatologic System

2

1. A 42-year-old woman presents to the clinic with worsening erythema, pain, and swelling of the right forearm, following an abrasion that occurred while gardening 2 days ago. In the past 12 hours, she has noticed a red streak extending up the arm from the abrasion site. What term describes this physical exam finding?

2. A 72-year-old man presents to the clinic with tense blisters and erosions on the abdomen and arms. He reports hives prior to the development of blisters. What laboratory test, obtained by a skin biopsy, will confirm the most likely diagnosis?

3. A 34-year-old woman presents to the clinic with erythema, papules, and pustules without comedones to the cheeks, nose, and chin. Her condition flares in sunlight, with consumption of spicy foods and extremes in temperature. What is the most likely diagnosis?

4. What is the recommended topical treatment for scabies?

5. What is the most important prognostic factor for malignant melanoma?

6. A 25-year-old man presents to the urgent care with severe pruritus and a rash to his lower extremities following a camping trip in the woods. On physical exam, he has multiple vesicles and bullae in linear patterns on the lower legs. Other members of his group are experiencing similar symptoms. What is the most appropriate treatment for the presumptive diagnosis?

7. An 11-year-old boy with well-controlled type 1 diabetes presents to the clinic with a slow onset of progressive skin hypopigmentation on the face, hands, and feet. The clinician determines that the depigmentation is due to an autoimmune process affecting melanocytes. What is the most likely diagnosis?

(See answers next page.)

1. Lymphangitis
The red streak represents lymphatic involvement and expansion of the infection.
Blueprint Task: History Taking and Performing Physical Examination
Cognitive Level: Apply

2. Histology and direct immunofluorescence microscopy
The clinical vignette supports the diagnosis of bullous pemphigoid. Serum for indirect immunofluorescence microscopy is also beneficial.
Blueprint Task: Using Diagnostic and Laboratory Studies
Cognitive Level: Analyze

3. Rosacea
Potential triggers for rosacea include environmental, dietary, and hormonal factors.
Blueprint Task: Formulating Most Likely Diagnosis
Cognitive Level: Apply

4. Scabicide such as permethrin 5%
Blueprint Task: Pharmaceutical Therapeutics
Cognitive Level: Recall

5. Depth
The ABCDEs (A: Asymmetry, B: Border irregularity, C: Color variation; D: Diameter > 6mm, E: Evolution) of melanoma are used in the initial assessment of risk in a patient with an atypical nevus to determine the need for biopsy.
Blueprint Task: Applying Basic Scientific Concepts
Cognitive Level: Apply

6. Topical corticosteroids
The clinical vignette supports the diagnosis of poison ivy contact dermatitis. Based on the location and isolated symptoms, high-potency topical corticosteroids are favored. Oral steroids are recommended for more diffuse, severe symptoms.
Blueprint Task: Clinical Intervention
Cognitive Level: Analyze

7. Vitiligo
Patients with vitiligo may have other autoimmune conditions. Genetic and environmental factors contribute to vitiligo.
Blueprint Task: Formulating Most Likely Diagnosis
Cognitive Level: Apply

8. What dermatologic condition presents as salmon-colored plaques with silvery scales, commonly found on the extensor surfaces of knees and elbows, seen in the following photo?

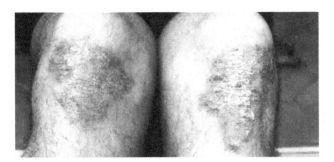

9. A 27-year-old man presents with a deep laceration of the left forearm following a wood-chipping accident. Why are radiographs insufficient in the evaluation of a foreign body in the wound?

10. A 40-year-old man presents to the emergency department with swelling, fluctuance, and tenderness at the gluteal cleft. What is the most appropriate treatment based on the presumptive diagnosis?

11. What term describes the development of lesions in areas of trauma, common in conditions such as lichen planus and psoriasis?

12. A 23-year-old woman with hypothyroidism and a BMI of 34 kg/m^2 presents to the clinic with frequently recurrent, painful, subcutaneous nodules and sinus tracts with scarring in the axillary and anogenital areas. She smokes socially and denies alcohol use. In addition to wound care, what two lifestyle modifications may help reduce symptoms?

13. A 33-year-old man presents to the clinic for his annual physical. He has no known prior health issues. Physical exam reveals symmetric brown papillomatous and velvety cutaneous thickening over the posterolateral neck and bilateral axilla. The patient should be screened for what underlying medical condition?

14. A healthy 10-year-old child presents to the clinic with lesions on the trunk, upper arms, and neck that do not tan. Physical exam reveals scattered macules varying in color, including pink, tan, and white. What class of medication is recommended for the most likely diagnosis?

15. The clinician applies gentle pressure laterally to unaffected skin in a patient with pemphigus vulgaris. Skin sloughing occurs due to fragility of the bullae. What is the name of this sign?

(See answers next page.)

8. Psoriasis
Blueprint Task: *History Taking and Performing Physical Examination*
Cognitive Level: *Recall*

9. Wood is radiolucent
Imaging modalities such as ultrasound, CT, or MRI are necessary to assess for the presence of a wooden foreign body.
Blueprint Task: *Using Diagnostic and Laboratory Studies*
Cognitive Level: *Apply*

10. Incision and drainage
The clinical vignette supports the diagnosis of pilonidal abscess.
Blueprint Task: *Clinical Intervention*
Cognitive Level: *Apply*

11. Koebner phenomenon
Blueprint Task: *Applying Basic Scientific Concepts*
Cognitive Level: *Recall*

12. Smoking cessation and weight management
The clinical vignette supports the diagnosis of hidradenitis suppurativa.
Blueprint Task: *Health Maintenance, Patient Education, and Preventive Measures*
Cognitive Level: *Analyze*

13. Diabetes mellitus
The clinical vignette describes acanthosis nigricans, which is frequently associated with insulin resistance.
Blueprint Task: *Formulating Most Likely Diagnosis*
Cognitive Level: *Apply*

14. Antifungal
The clinical vignette supports the diagnosis of tinea versicolor caused by the *Malassezia* species. Topical antifungal treatments include selenium sulfide lotion and ketoconazole shampoo. Systemic antifungal therapy may be used, however, it is not typically first-line in children.
Blueprint Task: *Pharmaceutical Therapeutics*
Cognitive Level: *Analyze*

15. Nikolsky sign
Blueprint Task: *Applying Basic Scientific Concepts*
Cognitive Level: *Recall*

16. A 67-year-old woman presents to the clinic for evaluation of an asymptomatic pigmented lesion on the back, as seen in the following photo. She denies pain, bleeding, or recent changes in size or color. What is the most appropriate treatment recommendation based on the presumptive diagnosis?

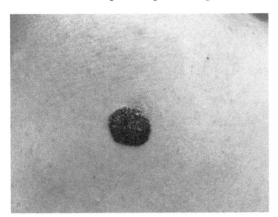

17. Sun exposure is the most important modifiable risk factor in the development of melanoma. In addition to using sun protection factor (SPF) sunscreen and protective clothing, what other specific sun safety counseling should be recommended?

18. A 25-year-old woman presents to the emergency department two weeks after starting trimethoprim-sulfamethoxazole for a urinary tract infection. She reports fever, dysphagia, dysuria, and burning of her eyes. Physical exam reveals mucocutaneous lesions. What other dermatologic finding is commonly associated with the presumptive diagnosis?

19. A 54-year-old man with a history of AIDS and paraplegia is admitted from the long-term center to the hospital with a stage 4 decubitus pressure injury. Patient was advised on wound care management and optimizing nutrition status. What other clinical intervention may aid in preventing recurrent pressure injuries in this high-risk patient?

20. What is the most common dermatophytosis caused by *Trichophyton rubrum*?

21. An 82-year-old man with type 2 diabetes and visual impairment presents to the clinic with a rash on the lower legs for the last two weeks. On physical exam, "punched out" ulcers with overlying crusts resembling cigarette burns are present on the lower legs. What is the most likely diagnosis?

22. When initiating treatment with isotretinoin for acne vulgaris, what baseline labs should be ordered?

23. What term describes a well-circumscribed, erythematous, tender nodule arising from an inflamed hair follicle?

(See answers next page.)

16. No treatment is necessary

The clinical vignette supports the diagnosis of seborrheic keratosis (SK). SK typically presents with a roughened, stuck-on appearance. Clinical intervention, such as cryotherapy, may be considered if symptomatic or cosmetic concerns.

Blueprint Task: Clinical Intervention
Cognitive Level: Analyze

17. Avoid peak ultraviolet (UV) B hours

Blueprint Task: Health Maintenance, Patient Education, and Preventive Measures
Cognitive Level: Recall

18. Atypical target lesion

The clinical vignette supports the diagnosis of Stevens-Johnson Syndrome (SJS). Early SJS presents with eruption of dark red macules that coalesce and may progress to complete epidermal detachment.

Blueprint Task: History Taking and Performing Physical Examination
Cognitive Level: Analyze

19. Pressure reducing devices

Immobility and immunocompromised state are risk factors for developing pressure injury and secondary infection.

Blueprint Task: Clinical Intervention
Cognitive Level: Apply

20. Tinea pedis

Blueprint Task: Applying Basic Scientific Concepts
Cognitive Level: Recall

21. Ecthyma

Ecthyma is a form of impetigo that is more common in the elderly and characteristically demonstrates ulcers. Poor hygiene increases the risk.

Blueprint Task: Formulating Most Likely Diagnosis
Cognitive Level: Apply

22. CBC, liver tests, lipid panel, and pregnancy test in females

Serum triglycerides should be repeated at 4 and 8 weeks. Females are also required to have a negative pregnancy test before starting the medication and repeated monthly.

Blueprint Task: Using Diagnostic and Laboratory Studies
Cognitive Level: Apply

23. Furuncle

Blueprint Task: History Taking and Performing Physical Examination
Cognitive Level: Recall

24. A 30-year-old woman is diagnosed with cellulitis that can effectively be treated outpatient. After providing emergency department precautions, what can the clinician demonstrate and advise the patient to perform at home to monitor progression?

25. A 24-year-old healthy woman develops scattered pustules and papules on both legs after spending an evening in a hot tub. The rash is mildly pruritic but not painful. What clinical intervention should be recommended?

26. A 35-year-old woman with no known medical conditions presents to the clinic with hair loss. Physical exam reveals thinning of the hair at the vertex of the scalp. What treatment is recommended for the presumptive diagnosis?

27. What is the typical physical exam finding associated with molluscum contagiosum?

28. A 47-year-old man with a moderately large, mobile, non-tender neck mass undergoes an MRI with contrast. What finding would be most indicative of a lipoma on T1 weighted image?

(See answers next page.)

24. Mark the borders

Expansive areas of redness represent worsening infection. Serial marking allows for the comparison of interval change.

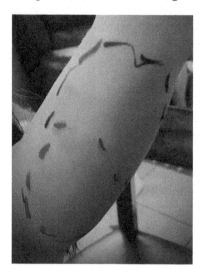

Blueprint Task: Health Maintenance, Patient Education, and Preventive Measures
Cognitive Level: Apply

25. No treatment is necessary

The clinical vignette supports the diagnosis of hot-tub folliculitis. This rash is typically self-limited and resolves within 2 weeks.
Blueprint Task: Clinical Intervention
Cognitive Level: Analyze

26. Minoxidil 5%

The clinical vignette supports the diagnosis of androgenetic alopecia in a premenopausal woman.
Blueprint Task: Pharmaceutical Therapeutics
Cognitive Level: Analyze

27. Umbilicated dome-shaped papule

Blueprint Task: History Taking and Performing Physical Examination
Cognitive Level: Recall

28. Bright appearing mass

Fat/air density appears brighter on T1 weighted images.
Blueprint Task: Using Diagnostic and Laboratory Studies
Cognitive Level: Apply

29. A 72-year-old man with type 2 diabetes presents to the clinic with a 2-day history of worsening fever, chills, and a painful erythematous facial rash. He is febrile at 38.3°C (101°F). Physical exam reveals well-defined, edematous areas of erythema over the cheeks and nose. What is the most likely diagnosis?

30. A child with known fungal scalp dermatitis develops a boggy, swollen, painful plaque. What term describes this dermatologic finding?

31. A 76-year-old woman presents with severe shooting pain followed by a vesicular rash along the right side of her trunk in a dermatomal pattern. When would the initiation of antivirals be most effective?

32. A 34-year-old woman presents with progressively worsening pain in her right index finger since acrylic nail application two weeks ago. Physical exam shows erythema, tenderness, and swelling at the lateral aspect of the nail fold without fluctuance. She has attempted warm soaks and elevation with minimal improvement. What is the most appropriate next step in the management of the presumptive diagnosis?

33. A 63-year-old man presents with a slow-growing papule on his left cheek. The papule is pearly translucent with rolled borders and telangiectasias. What is the most likely diagnosis?

34. Burrow lesions and excoriations in the interdigital webs, fingers, wrists, and axillae are pathognomonic for what condition?

35. A 27-year-old man develops a painful grouping of vesicles with an erythematous base on the penile shaft after sexual activity with a new partner. While the history and physical exam alone supports the presumptive diagnosis, what laboratory testing is preferred to confirm the diagnosis?

36. What medication most commonly induces bullous pemphigoid?

(See answers next page.)

29. Erysipelas

Erysipelas is known for sharply demarcated borders, while typical cellulitis may have ill-defined borders of erythema. Fever is more common with erysipelas than with typical cellulitis.

Blueprint Task: Formulating Most Likely Diagnosis
Cognitive Level: Apply

30. Kerion

Blueprint Task: Applying Basic Scientific Concepts
Cognitive Level: Recall

31. Within 72 hours of rash onset

The clinical vignette supports the diagnosis of herpes zoster. Timely antiviral treatment shortens the course, minimizes symptoms, and prevents chronic symptoms.

Blueprint Task: Pharmaceutical Therapeutics
Cognitive Level: Apply

32. Antibiotics

The clinical vignette supports the diagnosis of paronychia. Incision and drainage will be required if abscess is present.

Blueprint Task: Clinical Intervention
Cognitive Level: Analyze

33. Basal cell carcinoma (BCC)

BCC is the most common skin cancer and is found on sun exposed areas, including the face and head.

Blueprint Task: Formulating Most Likely Diagnosis
Cognitive Level: Apply

34. Scabies

Blueprint Task: History Taking and Performing Physical Examination
Cognitive Level: Recall

35. PCR assay

The clinical vignette supports the diagnosis of herpes simplex virus (HSV) infection. The laboratory evaluation varies based on clinical presentation. Viral culture may be used if vesicles are still present. PCR and viral culture include HSV-1 and HSV-2 typing.

Blueprint Task: Using Diagnostic and Laboratory Studies
Cognitive Level: Analyze

36. Furosemide

Blueprint Task: Pharmaceutical Therapeutics
Cognitive Level: Recall

37. A 27-year-old healthy woman presents to the clinic with a minimally pruritic rash. She developed a 3 cm macular eruption on the trunk 5 days ago. After developing the first lesion, she developed new smaller eruptions. Physical exam reveals macular lesions following the lines of cleavage. She denies sore throat, fever, or other symptoms. What is the recommended treatment for this patient?

38. A 56-year-old man with a history of squamous cell carcinoma presents to the clinic with a round, flesh-colored nodule with a crater-like center and keratin plug. The lesion has rapidly grown over the last 6 weeks. What is the most appropriate clinical intervention?

39. What dermatologic presentation classically proceeds a diffuse lacy, erythematous body rash in erythema infectiosum?

40. A 23-year-old man presents with a small growth on his heel and tenderness with walking. Physical exam reveals a small palpable mass with thick overlying callous formation. What technique may be used to confirm the diagnosis and may also aid in treatment?

41. What characteristic facial rash is associated with systemic lupus erythematosus?

42. Treatment is typically recommended for an actinic keratosis to prevent progression to what type of skin cancer?

43. A 34-year-old hairdresser presents to the clinic with a sudden onset of intensely pruritic, "tapioca-like" vesicles on the hands and between the fingers. She recalls similar but milder episodes in the past. She has tried avoiding irritants and using emollients without improvement. What would be the next step in the management of the presumptive diagnosis?

44. A 39-year-old man presents to the clinic for treatment of his toenail. He describes yellowing and thickening of the nail over the last year, as seen in the following photo. What is the most effective treatment for this condition?

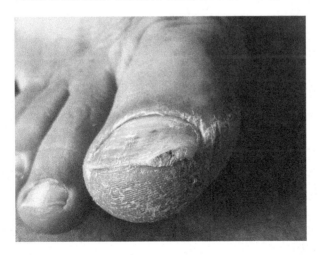

(See answers next page.)

37. No treatment is necessary

The clinical vignette supports the diagnosis of pityriasis rosea, which is typically self-limited. The initial macular eruption describes the herald patch followed by the "Christmas tree" or "fir tree" patterned rash, which may persist a few months. Pharmacologic treatment is reserved for more severe cases.

Blueprint Task: Health Maintenance, Patient Education, and Preventive Measures
Cognitive Level: Analyze

38. Biopsy

The clinical vignette supports the diagnosis of keratoacanthoma.

Blueprint Task: Clinical Intervention
Cognitive Level: Analyze

39. Erythematous cheeks

Erythema infectiosum (fifth disease) is caused by parvovirus B-19. Erythematous cheeks are commonly referred to as a "slapped cheek" appearance.

Blueprint Task: History Taking and Performing Physical Examination
Cognitive Level: Apply

40. Paring

Paring the surface of the wart facilitates the clinical diagnosis of a verruca vulgaris (plantar wart) by revealing thrombosed capillaries often referred to as "seeds." Paring prior to cryotherapy is also shown to improve cure rates for plantar warts.

Blueprint Task: Using Diagnostic and Laboratory Studies
Cognitive Level: Apply

41. Malar (butterfly) rash

Blueprint Task: Formulating Most Likely Diagnosis
Cognitive Level: Recall

42. Squamous cell carcinoma

Blueprint Task: Health Maintenance, Patient Education, and Preventative Measures
Cognitive Level: Recall

43. Topical corticosteroids

The clinical vignette supports the diagnosis of dyshidrotic eczema. Excessive handwashing or chemical exposures increase the risk for this condition.

Blueprint Task: Pharmaceutical Therapeutics
Cognitive Level: Analyze

44. Oral terbinafine

The clinical vignette supports the diagnosis of onychomycosis. Oral antifungals are recommended when the nail matrix is involved. Terbinafine has shown to have a higher efficacy than itraconazole.

Blueprint Task: Pharmaceutical Therapeutics
Cognitive Level: Analyze

45. An 8-year-old boy is brought into the clinic by his pregnant mother for a pruritic rash starting on the head and spreading to the trunk. Prior to the rash, the patient had a low-grade fever with malaise and anorexia. Physical exam reveals clusters of papules, vesicles, erosions, and crusts in various stages of evolution. What condition is the mother's fetus potentially at risk for based on the presumptive diagnosis?

46. A 45-year-old man presents to the emergency department after sustaining a boiling water injury with burns to the torso and left arm. On physical exam, the skin is red, moist, and tender with blistering. What is the classification for the depth of this burn?

47. A 12-year-old girl with a past medical history of eczema presents to the clinic with long-standing bumps on the upper outer arms. Mother has a similar chronic rash. Physical exam reveals non-tender, rough, raised papules. What is the pathophysiology for the most likely diagnosis?

48. An 8-year-old girl is brought to the clinic after her mother noted her scratching her head excessively due to generalized pruritis of the area. She recently shared a comb with a classmate. What would be the expected physical exam findings based on the presumptive diagnosis?

(See answers next page.)

45. Congenital varicella-zoster virus (VZV) syndrome

The clinical vignette supports the diagnosis of varicella (chickenpox). If the mother does not have immunity to VZV, she should avoid contact with her son.

Blueprint Task: *Formulating Most Likely Diagnosis*
Cognitive Level: *Analyze*

46. Superficial partial thickness

In a superficial partial thickness burn, the epidermis and the superficial dermis are damaged, while the deeper layers of the dermis are spared. The Rule of Nines would also be used to calculate the body surface area involved.

Blueprint Task: *History Taking and Performing Physical Examination*
Cognitive Level: *Apply*

47. Keratinization of hair follicles

The clinical vignette supports the diagnosis of keratosis pilaris. Family history is helpful since this is an autosomal dominant, genetic condition.

Blueprint Task: *Formulating Most Likely Diagnosis*
Cognitive Level: *Analyze*

48. Lice and nits

The student has *Pediculus humanus capitis* (head lice), which is more common among school-aged children. Live mites or nits are frequently found at the shaft of the hair around the nape of the neck and/or the ears.

Blueprint Task: *History Taking and Performing Physical Examination*
Cognitive Level: *Apply*

Endocrine System

1. What condition is associated with hypercalcemia and may manifest with abdominal cramps, constipation, bone pain, nephrolithiasis, and depression?

2. A 67-year-old man with type 2 diabetes mellitus and coronary artery disease presents to the emergency department with worsening weakness, fatigue, polyuria, and polydipsia over the past week. He was recently hospitalized for a myocardial infarction status post-revascularization. The patient appears lethargic with poor skin turgor. Labs reveal blood glucose level of 780 mg/dL and serum osmolality of 310 mOsm/kg with a normal serum pH and anion gap. There is no evidence of ketonemia. What is the presumptive diagnosis?

3. Which vitamin supplementation is recommended for exclusively breastfed newborns?

4. A 65-year-old man with a history of laryngeal cancer status post-radiation therapy presents to the clinic with neck pain and dysphagia. Physical exam reveals a palpable thyroid nodule. Ultrasound reveals a thyroid nodule that is >1 cm with microcalcifications, irregular margins, and extrathyroidal extension. What diagnostic procedure is most appropriate at this time?

5. What pharmacologic therapy is most appropriate in the treatment of central diabetes insipidus?

6. A 52-year-old patient with well-controlled hyperlipidemia presents to the clinic with gradual skin changes around the eyes. Physical exam reveals multiple raised, yellow non-tender plaques, as seen in the following photo. What term describes this physical exam finding?

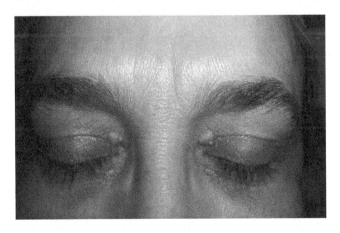

1. Primary hyperparathyroidism
The classic adage of "groans, bones, stones, and psychiatric overtones" is a constellation of symptoms associated with hypercalcemia seen in primary hyperparathyroidism.
Blueprint Task: *History Taking and Performing Physical Examination*
Cognitive Level: *Apply*

2. Hyperosmolar hyperglycemic state (HHS)
HHS generally presents in patients with type 2 diabetes mellitus. It is characterized by markedly elevated plasma glucose levels and serum osmolality in the absence of acidosis and ketonemia. Infection, myocardial infarction, stroke, or recent operation can precipitate HHS.
Blueprint Task: *Formulating Most Likely Diagnosis*
Cognitive Level: *Apply*

3. Vitamin D
Blueprint Task: *Health Maintenance, Patient Education, and Preventive Measures*
Cognitive Level: *Recall*

4. Ultrasound-guided fine-needle aspiration (FNA) biopsy
The patient's history of head-neck radiation therapy plus the sonographic features increases the risk of a malignant thyroid nodule.
Blueprint Task: *Clinical Intervention*
Cognitive Level: *Analyze*

5. Desmopressin
Blueprint Task: *Pharmaceutical Therapeutics*
Cognitive Level: *Recall*

6. Xanthelasma
Xanthelasma are well-circumscribed deposits of cholesterol that are usually located on the eyelids. This benign condition is frequently associated with dyslipidemia.
Blueprint Task: *History Taking and Performing Physical Examination*
Cognitive Level: *Apply*

7. A 73-year-old woman is status postsurgical removal of a parathyroid adenoma for primary hyperparathyroidism. She developed perioral numbness, carpopedal spasms, and muscle cramping. Physical exam reveals facial muscle contractions upon tapping the facial nerve. What is the expected laboratory abnormality?

8. Routine monofilament testing is recommended to screen for what potential microvascular complication of type 2 diabetes?

9. A 55-year-old man with type 2 diabetes mellitus managed with insulin lispro begins to develop a headache, heart palpitations, sweating, and tremulousness without confusion or loss of consciousness. His blood glucose is 61 mg/dL. What intervention is most appropriate in the management of this condition?

10. What condition results when excess growth hormone is secreted prior to closure of epiphyseal growth plates?

11. Which thionamide drug provides convenient dosing and is less likely to cause liver injury in Graves' hyperthyroidism?

12. Newborn screening for congenital hypothyroidism is necessary to prevent what primary complication if left untreated?

13. A 54-year-old man with a recent head injury presents with urinary frequency and polyuria. A 24-hour urine volume exceeds >8L. Urine osmolality is 70 mOsm/kg and serum osmolality is 310 mOsm/kg. Serum sodium is 160 mEq/L. A urine dipstick is negative for glucose. What is the most likely diagnosis?

14. A patient presents with symptoms of type 2 diabetes. When utilizing HbA1c, what is the minimum level required to confirm this diagnosis?

(See answers next page.)

7. Hypocalcemia

Hypocalcemia can transiently develop following parathyroid surgery. Chvostek sign describes the physical exam finding.
Blueprint Task: Using Diagnostic and Laboratory Studies
Cognitive Level: Analyze

8. Neuropathy

Blueprint Task: Health Maintenance, Patient Education, and Preventive Measures
Cognitive Level: Recall

9. Glucose

The patient is experiencing insulin-induced hypoglycemia. Blood glucose should be monitored closely.
Blueprint Task: Clinical Intervention
Cognitive Level: Analyze

10. Gigantism

Blueprint Task: Applying Basic Scientific Concepts
Cognitive Level: Recall

11. Methimazole

Methimazole is preferred over propylthiouracil (PTU) in the treatment of hyperthyroidism, except during the first trimester of pregnancy. Propranolol is also commonly prescribed for symptomatic relief.
Blueprint Task: Pharmaceutical Therapeutics
Cognitive Level: Apply

12. Neurocognitive impairment

Thyroid hormone is necessary for brain and growth development. Congenital hypothyroidism (cretinism) may also lead to short stature and other abnormalities.
Blueprint Task: Health Maintenance, Patient Education, and Preventive Measures
Cognitive Level: Apply

13. Diabetes insipidus

The clinical vignette supports the diagnosis of diabetes insipidus secondary to decreased release of antidiuretic hormone (ADH), which leads to abnormally large volumes of dilute urine. Common causes of diabetes insipidus include tumor, surgery, head injury, or illness resulting in damage to the hypothalamus or the pituitary gland.
Blueprint Task: Formulating Most Likely Diagnosis
Cognitive Level: Apply

14. 6.5%

Blueprint Task: Using Diagnostic and Laboratory Studies
Cognitive Level: Recall

15. A 33-year-old woman with a BMI of 33 kg/m² presents to the clinic with recurrent chronic candidal vulvovaginitis. What underlying condition should be suspected in this patient?

16. A 26-year-old man with a BMI of 23.2 kg/m² presents with a blood pressure of 147/96 mm Hg. He has a history of hypertension refractory to triple therapy along with hypokalemia managed with potassium chloride. What is the most likely diagnosis in this patient?

17. In a patient with high-risk thyroid cancer, what adjunct therapy is recommended following complete thyroidectomy?

18. What medication is most appropriate in the treatment of hypothyroidism?

19. What cells stimulate insulin release in response to high glucose?

20. A 54-year-old woman presents to the office to review her dual-energy x-ray absorptiometry (DXA) results. She denies chronic medical conditions. Social history reveals tobacco use of 20 pack-years and consumes 4-5 beers on the weekends. Her T-score is noted to be one standard deviation below peak bone mineral density. What specific type of exercise program is most beneficial for the presumptive diagnosis?

21. What sign, indicative of hypocalcemia, is demonstrated by inflating the sphygmomanometer to 20 mm Hg above the patient's systolic blood pressure for a duration of 3 minutes and observing for carpal spasm?

22. A 22-year-old man with a history of Hashimoto's thyroiditis presents to the clinic with several months of fatigue, weakness, nausea, weight loss, and lightheadedness upon standing. Physical exam reveals orthostatic hypotension and hyperpigmentation of the gums and skinfolds. Cortisol levels are decreased in the morning. What test confirms the presumptive diagnosis?

(See answers next page.)

15. Diabetes mellitus
Diabetes mellitus predisposes patients for infections, including fungal, and may be treatment resistant leading to recurrence.
Blueprint Task: *History Taking and Performing Physical Examination*
Cognitive Level: *Apply*

16. Hyperaldosteronism
Hyperaldosteronism should be considered in patients presenting with hypokalemia and refractory hypertension. Aldosterone aids in the regulation of sodium and potassium.
Blueprint Task: *Formulating Most Likely Diagnosis*
Cognitive Level: *Apply*

17. Radioiodine therapy
Since the thyroid gland absorbs the majority of iodine in the body, radioiodine targets the thyroid cells allowing the radiation to destroy any remaining thyroid tissue, including the cancer cells that may have migrated to lymph nodes or other areas in the body. Absolute contraindications for radioiodine therapy are pregnancy and breastfeeding.
Blueprint Task: *Clinical Intervention*
Cognitive Level: *Apply*

18. Synthetic thyroxine
Blueprint Task: *Pharmaceutical Therapeutics*
Cognitive Level: *Recall*

19. Pancreatic beta cells
Pancreatic beta cells respond to high glucose, whereas pancreatic alpha cells release glucagon in response to low glucose.
Blueprint Task: *Applying Basic Scientific Concepts*
Cognitive Level: *Apply*

20. Weight-bearing
The clinical vignette supports the diagnosis of osteoporosis. Discontinuation of alcohol and tobacco is recommended, and vitamin D supplementation should be considered.
Blueprint Task: *Clinical Intervention*
Cognitive Level: *Analyze*

21. Trousseau's sign
Blueprint Task: *History Taking and Performing Physical Examination*
Cognitive Level: *Recall*

22. Cosyntropin (ACTH) stimulation test
The clinical vignette supports the diagnosis of primary adrenal insufficiency.
Blueprint Task: *Using Diagnostic and Laboratory Studies*
Cognitive Level: *Analyze*

23. A 28-year-old man presents to the clinic with concerns about infertility. On physical exam, he has gynecomastia and small testes. Laboratory studies reveal a low free and total serum testosterone with a high LH and FSH. What underlying genetic condition should be considered?

24. A body mass index (BMI) of 25–29.9 kg/m^2 signifies what weight classification?

25. What commonly prescribed oral hypoglycemic medication may be associated with lactic acidosis?

26. Patients with diabetes require home blood glucose monitoring, blood pressure control, lipid management, and lifestyle modifications to prevent what major cardiovascular complication?

27. What class of oral hypoglycemic medication may cause fluid retention and worsen heart failure?

28. What would be the expected findings of parathyroid hormone (PTH), serum calcium, and serum phosphate in primary hyperparathyroidism?

29. What is the characteristic anatomic distribution of diabetic peripheral neuropathy?

30. A 35-year-old woman with a BMI of 35 kg/m^2 presents with amenorrhea for 6 months and inability to conceive. Physical exam reveals excessive acne on her face and back, along with hirsutism. Fasting blood glucose is 120 mg/dL. What is the most likely diagnosis?

(See answers next page.)

23. Klinefelter syndrome

Klinefelter syndrome represents a chromosomal abnormality, 47 XXY, resulting in hypogonadism, testicular dysfunction, infertility, and gynecomastia. Typically, this syndrome is not identified until adulthood when the patient struggles with infertility. Patients may still be able to father a child with assisted reproductive procedures.

Blueprint Task: Formulating Most Likely Diagnosis
Cognitive Level: Apply

24. Overweight

Blueprint Task: Applying Basic Scientific Concepts
Cognitive Level: Recall

25. Metformin

Blueprint Task: Pharmaceutical Therapeutics
Cognitive Level: Recall

26. Atherosclerotic cardiovascular disease (ASCVD)

ASCVD is the macrovascular complication of diabetes and can manifest as coronary heart disease, cerebrovascular disease, and/or peripheral arterial disease. Lifestyle modifications include nutritional therapy, physical activity, and weight loss if needed.

Blueprint Task: Health Maintenance, Patient Education, and Preventive Measures
Cognitive Level: Apply

27. Thiazolidinediones (TZDs)

Blueprint Task: Pharmaceutical Therapeutics
Cognitive Level: Recall

28. Elevated PTH, hypercalcemia, hypophosphatemia

In primary hyperparathyroidism, excess PTH is secreted, which causes increased calcium resorption from the bone and kidney, increased calcium uptake in the intestine, and increased phosphate excretion.

Blueprint Task: Using Diagnostic and Laboratory Studies
Cognitive Level: Apply

29. "Stocking and glove" in the extremities

Blueprint Task: History Taking and Performing Physical Examination
Cognitive Level: Recall

30. Polycystic ovarian syndrome

Patient education focused on weight loss, carbohydrate restriction, and exercise is essential and may induce ovulation and reverse metabolic changes.

Blueprint Task: Formulating Most Likely Diagnosis
Cognitive Level: Apply

31. A 40-year-old woman presents with increasing problems of paroxysmal attacks of headaches, sweating, elevated blood pressure, and palpitations that last about 30 minutes. The episodes are increasing in frequency and severity over the last 12 months. The blood pressure elevation is unresponsive to trials of antihypertensive medication. 24-hour urinary metanephrines and catecholamines are significantly elevated. CT scan of the abdomen and pelvis is ordered to investigate for what presumptive diagnosis?

32. A 62-year-old man with hypertension and hyperlipidemia was recently diagnosed with type 2 diabetes. What laboratory assessment provides an average blood sugar over the previous 2 to 3 months?

33. A 33-year-old woman presents, following a recent viral upper respiratory illness, for neck pain and fatigue for the past few weeks. Physical exam reveals low-grade fever and a tender thyroid. Labs demonstrate elevated ESR and low thyroid antibody titers. What is the most appropriate treatment based on the presumptive diagnosis?

34. A 23-year-old man with a BMI of 31 kg/m², hyperglycemia, and hyperlipidemia has hyperpigmented velvety plaques on the posterior aspect of the neck, as shown in the following photo. What is the term for this dermatologic finding?

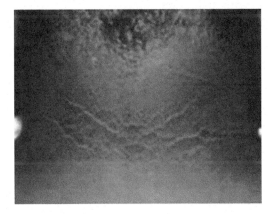

35. What class of medication is the mainstay therapy for micro- or macroprolactinomas?

36. Hyperparathyroidism, gastroenteropancreatic neuroendocrine tumors (GEP-NET), and pituitary adenomas comprise what endocrine disorder?

37. A 54-year-old sedentary woman presents with drenching night sweats that have disrupted sleep for the past 7 months. She reports worsening facial flushing, fatigue, decreased libido, and amenorrhea for over 1 year. What lifestyle modification may be beneficial in alleviating symptoms associated with the presumptive diagnosis?

(*See answers next page.*)

31. Pheochromocytoma

The clinical manifestations of a pheochromocytoma are caused by the secretion of epinephrine and norepinephrine. Classically, the detection of an adrenal mass with abnormal biochemical markers supports the diagnosis of a pheochromocytoma.
Blueprint Task: Using Diagnostic and Laboratory Studies
Cognitive Level: Analyze

32. HbA1c

Blueprint Task: Health Maintenance, Patient Education, and Preventive Measures
Cognitive Level: Recall

33. Nonsteroidal anti-inflammatory drug (NSAID)

The clinical vignette supports the diagnosis of subacute painful thyroiditis. NSAIDs including aspirin relieve pain and inflammation. Glucocorticoids may be given if a patient is unresponsive or has significant local or systemic symptoms.
Blueprint Task: Clinical Intervention
Cognitive Level: Analyze

34. Acanthosis nigricans

Acanthosis nigricans is frequently associated with insulin resistance.
Blueprint Task: History Taking and Performing Physical Examination
Cognitive Level: Apply

35. Oral dopamine agonists

Blueprint Task: Pharmaceutical Therapeutics
Cognitive Level: Recall

36. Multiple endocrine neoplasia (MEN) 1

Blueprint Task: Applying Basic Scientific Concepts
Cognitive Level: Recall

37. Regular exercise

The clinical vignette supports the diagnosis of menopause with vasomotor symptoms. Menopausal symptoms may improve with dietary changes, smoking cessation, and exercise.
Blueprint Task: Health Maintenance, Patient Education, and Preventive Measures
Cognitive Level: Apply

38. A 30-year-old man presents with a 6-month history of decreased libido and difficulty achieving and maintaining an erection. He has been tired, depressed, and has generalized thinning of his body hair. Physical exam reveals small testicles. Total serum testosterone, LH, and FSH are low. What is the most likely diagnosis?

39. A 56-year-old man with longstanding diabetes is overdue for his yearly diabetic retinopathy exam. Fundoscopic exam reveals new tortuous blood vessels arising from the disc and extending to the margins. What term describes these findings?

40. Angiotensin-converting enzyme inhibitors (ACE-I) and angiotensin receptor blockers (ARB) are commonly used in renal disease. What other class of medication may be used in the management of diabetes, albuminuria, and prevention of progression to end-stage kidney disease by reducing intraglomerular pressure?

41. Which hormones are released by the posterior pituitary?

42. A 65-year-old man with hypercholesteremia and a mechanical aortic valve replacement presents to the clinic requesting testosterone replacement therapy. Current medications include coumadin, atorvastatin, and ezetimibe. Labs reveal low serum testosterone. If testosterone is prescribed, what lab must be monitored in this patient in addition to serum testosterone?

43. What visual field finding is classically associated with a pituitary adenoma impinging the optic chiasm?

44. A 43-year-old woman with type 1 diabetes presents to the emergency department with nausea, vomiting, and abdominal pain for 2 days. She describes worsening dysuria, frequent urination, and increased thirst for the past several days. Physical exam reveals a blood pressure 100/70 mm Hg and heart rate 113 bpm with deep, rapid, labored breathing. Serum blood glucose is 457 mg/dL and sodium is 131 mEq/L with a metabolic acidosis and increased anion gap. Urine dipstick is positive for leukocyte esterase, nitrites, glucose, and ketones, consistent with a urinary tract infection (UTI). What emergent condition was precipitated by her infection?

45. A 54-year-old man with type 2 diabetes is prescribed injectable insulin therapy. What patient education should be provided to prevent lipohypertrophy?

(See answers next page.)

38. Hypogonadotropic hypogonadism

Hypogonadotropic hypogonadism presents with normal or low levels of LH and FSH, low total serum or free testosterone, and the characteristic findings as described in the vignette.

Blueprint Task: Formulating Most Likely Diagnosis

Cognitive Level: Analyze

39. Neovascularization

Neovascularization is caused by abnormal permeability and vascular occlusion in patients with diabetic retinopathy.

Blueprint Task: History Taking and Performing Physical Examination

Cognitive Level: Apply

40. Sodium-glucose co-transporter 2 inhibitors (SGLT2)

Blueprint Task: Pharmaceutical Therapeutics

Cognitive Level: Recall

41. Vasopressin and oxytocin

Blueprint Task: Applying Basic Scientific Concepts

Cognitive Level: Recall

42. International normalized ratio (INR)

The combination of coumadin and testosterone may result in an increased INR.

Blueprint Task: Clinical Intervention

Cognitive Level: Analyze

43. Bitemporal hemianopsia

Blueprint Task: History Taking and Performing Physical Examination

Cognitive Level: Recall

44. Diabetic ketoacidosis (DKA)

DKA is an acute complication of diabetes, occurring primarily in patients with type 1 diabetes, triggered by infection, trauma, or physiologic stress. Patients may present with polydipsia, polyuria, Kussmaul respirations, and fruity odor to breath.

Blueprint Task: Formulating Most Likely Diagnosis

Cognitive Level: Analyze

45. Rotation of injection sites

Lipohypertrophy, the accumulation of fat beneath the skin, may result from insulin being injected repeatedly in the same location. If a patient is on an insulin pump, the infusion site should also be rotated.

Blueprint Task: Health Maintenance, Patient Education, and Preventive Measures

Cognitive Level: Apply

46. What cardiac arrhythmia may be associated with excess thyroid hormone replacement requiring lower starting doses in the elderly?

47. What class of oral hypoglycemic medication stimulates beta-cell insulin release and may cause hypoglycemia and weight gain?

48. What syndrome presents as profound hypotonia in infancy followed by obsessive hyperphagia with weight gain in early childhood?

49. What would be the expected findings of parathyroid hormone (PTH), serum calcium, and serum phosphate in secondary hyperparathyroidism?

50. A 29-year-old woman with hyperthyroidism presents with proptosis, lid retraction, and lid lag. What condition describes the autoimmune process affecting the retroocular tissue causing the ophthalmologic findings?

51. Late-night salivary cortisol and 24-hour urinary free cortisol secretion are valuable in the initial evaluation of Cushing's syndrome. What additional first-line laboratory test may be utilized to diagnose Cushing's syndrome?

52. A 64-year-old woman with poorly controlled diabetes presents with nausea, vomiting, and early satiety. There are no signs of small bowel or mechanical gastric outlet obstruction. Gastric emptying scintigraphy reveals delayed emptying of both liquids and solids. Which two classes of medication may provide this patient relief?

53. What type of thyroid carcinoma is the most common and typically grows slowly, spreads locally, and is generally the least aggressive?

54. A 4-year-old girl presents as a new patient and is noted to have short fourth metacarpals, low-set ears, wide-spaced nipples, and a webbed neck. She has a bicuspid aortic valve. Based on the presumptive diagnosis, what clinical intervention may help prevent excessively short stature in this child?

(*See answers next page.*)

46. Atrial fibrillation

A lower initial starting dose of thyroid hormone replacement is also recommended in patients with increased cardiac demand.

Blueprint Task: Clinical Intervention
Cognitive Level: Apply

47. Sulfonylureas

Blueprint Task: Pharmaceutical Therapeutics
Cognitive Level: Recall

48. Prader–Willi syndrome (PWS)

PWS results from chromosomal abnormalities affecting genes on chromosome 15, leading to growth hormone deficiency. Obsessive hyperphagia is the hallmark finding with this syndrome.

Blueprint Task: Formulating Most Likely Diagnosis
Cognitive Level: Apply

49. Elevated PTH, hypocalcemia, and hyperphosphatemia

In secondary hyperparathyroidism, PTH levels are elevated in response to chronic hypocalcemia. The most common causes of secondary hyperparathyroidism are vitamin D deficiency and chronic kidney disease, which may contribute to hyperphosphatemia.

Blueprint Task: Using Diagnostic and Laboratory Studies
Cognitive Level: Apply

50. Graves' orbitopathy

Blueprint Task: History Taking and Performing Physical Examination
Cognitive Level: Recall

51. Dexamethasone suppression test

Selection of one or more diagnostic tests is based on the index of suspicion for Cushing's syndrome. These laboratory tests assess for inappropriate secretion of cortisol.

Blueprint Task: Clinical Intervention
Cognitive Level: Apply

52. Antiemetics and promotility agents

The clinical vignette supports the diagnosis of diabetic gastroparesis.

Blueprint Task: Pharmaceutical Therapeutics
Cognitive Level: Apply

53. Papillary thyroid carcinoma

Blueprint Task: Applying Basic Scientific Concepts
Cognitive Level: Recall

54. Recombinant growth hormone

The clinical vignette supports the diagnosis of Turner syndrome.

Blueprint Task: Clinical Intervention
Cognitive Level: Analyze

55. A 33-year-old woman presents to the clinic with anxiety, palpitations, weight loss, and frequent bowel movements. Physical exam reveals warm moist skin, tachycardia, proptosis, and an enlarged thyroid. She has a low TSH, elevated T4 and T3, and diffuse uptake on a radioactive iodine uptake scan. What is the most likely diagnosis?

56. What type of sodium disorder is anticipated in a patient with syndrome of inappropriate antidiuretic hormone (SIADH) secondary to small cell carcinoma of the lung?

57. What type of diabetic retinopathy is associated with microaneurysms, retinal hemorrhages, hard exudates, and cotton wool spots?

58. A 44-year-old woman presents to the clinic with fatigue, constipation, and weight gain. Physical exam reveals bradycardia, dry skin, and an enlarged thyroid. She has elevated TSH, low free T4, with thyroid peroxidase and thyroglobulin antibodies. What is the most likely diagnosis?

59. What is the most important initial intervention in the treatment of diabetic ketoacidosis (DKA)?

60. A 35-year-old man presents to the clinic stating that his ring no longer fits and his shoe size has increased gradually over the past few years. He was recently diagnosed with diabetes and hypertension. Labs reveal elevated serum insulin-like growth factor (IGF-1). What is the most likely diagnosis based on the physical exam findings in the following photo?

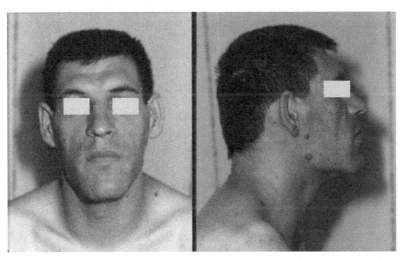

61. Which two types of insulin are appropriate as basal therapies to suppress hepatic glucose production?

(See answers next page.)

55. Hyperthyroidism

The clinical vignette supports the diagnosis of hyperthyroidism likely secondary to Graves' disease.

Blueprint Task: Formulating Most Likely Diagnosis
Cognitive Level: Apply

56. Hyponatremia

In SIADH, antidiuretic hormone (ADH) is secreted in the absence of a physiologic stimuli such as decreased effective circulating volume leading to hyponatremia.

Blueprint Task: Using Diagnostic and Laboratory Studies
Cognitive Level: Apply

57. Nonproliferative

Blueprint Task: History Taking and Performing Physical Examination
Cognitive Level: Recall

58. Hashimoto's thyroiditis

Hashimoto's thyroiditis is the most common cause of hypothyroidism in the United States.

Blueprint Task: Formulating Most Likely Diagnosis
Cognitive Level: Apply

59. Resuscitation with IV fluids

Patients with DKA are dehydrated and need aggressive fluid resuscitation to help improve the hyperglycemic and metabolic abnormalities associated with this condition. Immediately after initiation of fluid replacement, regular insulin should be given.

Blueprint Task: Clinical Intervention
Cognitive Level: Apply

60. Acromegaly

The classic presentation of acromegaly includes enlarged facial features such as protruding mandible, frontal bossing, thickening of the lips, enlarged nose, and prominent brows. Patients may also present with enlarged hands and feet, thickened skin, and other abnormalities on physical exam.

Blueprint Task: History Taking and Performing Physical Examination
Cognitive Level: Apply

61. Intermediate or long-acting insulin

Intermediate and long-acting insulin provide basal glucose control, whereas rapid-acting and short-acting regular insulin provide bolus control to cover carbohydrate intake at meals.

Blueprint Task: Pharmaceutical Therapeutics
Cognitive Level: Apply

62. A mother brings her 8-year-old daughter to the clinic for cyclical vaginal bleeding that has occurred over the past 3 months. Physical exam reveals no breast development or presence of pubic hair. She denies history of acne, body odor, or exposure to estradiol. Lab reveals the estradiol level to be within prepubertal range for females. What is the most likely diagnosis?

63. Referral to an ophthalmologist for patients with type 2 diabetes is required to assess for what condition?

64. A 33-year-old woman presents to the clinic with amenorrhea, infertility, and galactorrhea. She takes no medications. What is the primary laboratory test utilized in the evaluation of the presumptive diagnosis?

65. Aldosterone, cortisol, dehydroepiandrosterone (DHEA), and catecholamines are produced by what gland?

66. A 54-year-old woman presents to the clinic with fatigue, headaches, and weight gain. Physical exam reveals a blood pressure of 147/93 mm Hg, central obesity, abdominal striae, rounded face, and hirsutism. Random blood glucose is 190 mg/dL. What is the presumptive diagnosis?

(*See answers next page.*)

62. Premature menarche

Premature menarche presents with an earlier than expected onset of cyclical bleeding in the absence of secondary sexual characteristics.

Blueprint Task: *Formulating Most Likely Diagnosis*
Cognitive Level: *Apply*

63. Diabetic retinopathy

Blueprint Task: *History Taking and Performing Physical Examination*
Cognitive Level: *Recall*

64. Serum prolactin

The clinical vignette supports the diagnosis of hyperprolactinemia. Multiple factors may influence the prolactin level, and repeat testing may be needed.

Blueprint Task: *Using Diagnostic and Laboratory Studies*
Cognitive Level: *Apply*

65. Adrenal gland

Blueprint Task: *Applying Basic Scientific Concepts*
Cognitive Level: *Recall*

66. Cushing's syndrome

Cushing's syndrome results from increased cortisol secretion, generally from an adrenal tumor or excess exogenous glucocorticoid.

Blueprint Task: *Formulating Most Likely Diagnosis*
Cognitive Level: *Apply*

Eyes, Ears, Nose, and Throat

1. A 72-year-old patient presents to the clinic with hearing loss in the right ear. On physical exam, the Weber test lateralizes to the right side, and the Rinne test reveals bone conduction greater than air conduction. What type of hearing loss is most likely?

2. A 12-year-old boy presents to the clinic with a 6-day history of sore throat, fatigue, and fever of 38.9°C (102°F). Physical exam reveals erythema and enlargement of the tonsils with bilateral exudate and tender anterior and posterior cervical lymphadenopathy. Strep screen is negative and the heterophile agglutination test is positive. What would be the expected result of a peripheral blood smear?

3. A 22-year-old man presents to the clinic with an acute 1-day history of pain and foreign body sensation to the left eye. Fluorescein stain of the left eye reveals a dendritic pattern. What is the most likely diagnosis?

4. What antibiotic is recommended in a 6-year-old patient with recurrent acute otitis media resistant to amoxicillin?

5. A 45-year-old man with allergic rhinitis reports long-standing daily use of a topical nasal decongestant. The nasal congestion seems to be worse if he goes a few days without the topical decongestant. The clinician explains the dangers of consistent use greater than 5 consecutive days to avoid developing what condition?

6. A 72-year-old man presents to the clinic upon recommendation by the oral hygienist to evaluate white patches on the buccal mucosa. The patient has used chewing tobacco for 50 years. The white patches cannot be scraped off with a tongue blade. What clinical intervention is recommended?

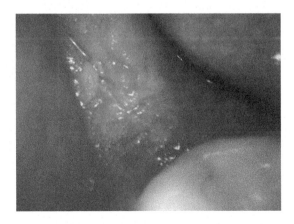

1. Conductive right-sided hearing loss

Weber and Rinne tests are used to evaluate patients with hearing loss and differentiate between conductive and sensorineural loss. With conductive hearing loss, the Weber test lateralizes to the impaired ear, and the Rinne test reveals bone conduction greater than air conduction on the affected side.

Blueprint Task: History Taking and Performing Physical Examination

Cognitive Level: Apply

2. Atypical lymphocytes

The clinical vignette supports the diagnosis of mononucleosis caused by the Epstein-Barr virus.

Blueprint Task: Using Diagnostic and Laboratory Studies

Cognitive Level: Analyze

3. Herpes simplex keratitis

Dendritic pattern is a classic finding in herpes keratitis defined as a branching tree-like figure.

Blueprint Task: Formulating Most Likely Diagnosis

Cognitive Level: Apply

4. Amoxicillin-clavulanate

Blueprint Task: Pharmaceutical Therapeutics

Cognitive Level: Recall

5. Rhinitis medicamentosa

Topical nasal decongestant use should be limited to no greater than 5 consecutive days to decrease the risk of rebound congestion. First-line medication for allergic rhinitis is topical nasal glucocorticoids.

Blueprint Task: Health Maintenance, Patient Education, and Preventive Measures

Cognitive Level: Apply

6. Biopsy

The clinical vignette supports the diagnosis of leukoplakia. Leukoplakia is associated with an increased risk of oral cancer, especially with a history of long-standing tobacco use.

Blueprint Task: Clinical Intervention

Cognitive Level: Apply

7. A 69-year-old man presents to the clinic with acute onset of unilateral blurred vision, halo, and eye pain. Physical exam reveals a fixed pupil, steamy cornea, and a firm globe. What specialized exam confirms the most likely diagnosis?

8. What is the most common organism associated with sialadenitis?

9. An 81-year-old man with a history of type 2 diabetes presents to the emergency department with fever and severe worsening left ear pain accompanied by purulent discharge. Antibiotic drops prescribed two days ago were ineffective. What is the best initial imaging study to evaluate for the presumptive diagnosis?

10. What ocular exam is recommended to monitor for progressive visual changes in patients with macular degeneration?

11. A 32-year-old woman presents to the clinic with vertigo. Physical exam reveals rhythmic, regular, slow drift of the eyes in one direction with a corrective jerk in the opposite direction. What term describes this ocular movement?

12. A 73-year-old woman presents to the clinic with chronic nasal congestion, rhinorrhea, and a postnasal drip that increase with triggers such as perfume and cigarette smoke. She denies ocular symptoms or sneezing. She has been avoiding triggers. Aside from intranasal antihistamine spray and intranasal ipratropium, what other pharmacologic class may be considered in the management of the presumptive diagnosis?

13. A patient presents with an inferior wall blow-out fracture of the left eye. Physical exam of the left eye reveals inability to look upward. What extraocular muscle is entrapped?

14. A 33-year-old woman presents to the clinic with a 2-day history of pain, swelling, tenderness, and redness overlying the lacrimal sac. What is the first-line pharmacologic therapy for the presumptive diagnosis to avoid potential complications?

(See answers next page.)

7. Gonioscopy

The clinical vignette supports the diagnosis of acute angle-closure glaucoma. Gonioscopy will reveal a narrow chamber angle.

Blueprint Task: History Taking and Performing Physical Examination
Cognitive Level: Analyze

8. *Staphylococcus aureus*

Blueprint Task: Applying Basic Scientific Concepts
Cognitive Level: Recall

9. CT of temporal bone

The clinical vignette supports the diagnosis of left malignant otitis externa, more common in immunocompromised patients. The CT of temporal bone with contrast will evaluate for bone erosion. MRI may also be used for evaluation.

Blueprint Task: Using Diagnostic and Laboratory Studies
Cognitive Level: Analyze

10. Daily Amsler grid checks

This exam monitors for worsening of vision and metamorphopsia.

Blueprint Task: Health Maintenance, Patient Education, and Preventive Measures
Cognitive Level: Apply

11. Jerk nystagmus

Jerk nystagmus has a slow and fast phase as compared to pendulum nystagmus, which has no fast phase.

Blueprint Task: Formulating Most Likely Diagnosis
Cognitive Level: Apply

12. Intranasal corticosteroid

The clinical vignette supports the diagnosis of nonallergic rhinitis (vasomotor rhinitis).

Blueprint Task: Pharmaceutical Therapeutics
Cognitive Level: Apply

13. Inferior rectus

Blueprint Task: Applying Basic Scientific Concepts
Cognitive Level: Recall

14. Empiric systemic antibiotic therapy

The clinical vignette supports the diagnosis of dacryocystitis. Empiric antibiotic therapy is started while awaiting culture. Potential complications of dacryocystitis include preseptal cellulitis, orbital cellulitis, and meningitis.

Blueprint Task: Clinical Intervention
Cognitive Level: Analyze

15. A 21-year-old man presents to the clinic with a chronic, slowly growing firm lump on the hard palate. He denies pain, dysphagia, difficulty chewing, or other problems. Physical exam reveals findings demonstrated in the following photo. What is the presumptive diagnosis?

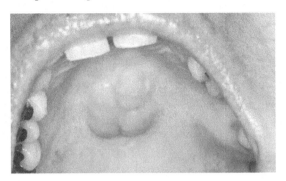

16. A 17-year-old football player presents to the clinic with a slight hearing loss over the last two weeks after sustaining a contusion to the left side of the head during a tackle. He denies loss of consciousness. Physical exam reveals a left tympanic membrane (TM) perforation. What would be the expected tympanogram result due to the perforation?

17. By what age does the American Academy of Pediatric Dentistry and American Academy of Pediatrics recommend all children have a dental caries-risk assessment by a health-care provider?

18. A 30-year-old woman presents to the clinic with acute pain and decreased vision in her right eye. An ocular exam reveals a mid-dilated pupil on the right, which is poorly responsive to light, and a shadow on the nasal side of the iris. What intravenous pharmacologic therapy may be utilized for the presumptive diagnosis?

19. An 82-year-old man presents to the clinic with a slowly progressive, triangular thickening spreading across the right cornea. He denies eye pain or change in vision. The clinician refers the patient to ophthalmology for evaluation for this potentially sight-threatening condition. What is the most likely diagnosis?

20. A 25-year-old healthy woman reports seasonal issues with rhinorrhea and sneezing since moving to the Midwest. Occasional doses of over-the-counter antihistamines improved symptoms; however, she dislikes oral medications. What is the recommended pharmacologic therapy for the presumptive diagnosis?

21. What vascular network is most commonly involved in epistaxis?

22. A 4-year-old girl presents to the emergency department with fever, neck pain, and dysphagia. What initial imaging should be performed to evaluate for retropharyngeal infection in a patient without airway compromise?

(See answers next page.)

15. Torus palatinus

Torus palatinus is an asymptomatic, common bony growth on the hard palate. The bony growth typically begins during childhood and slowly enlarges.

Blueprint Task: History Taking and Performing Physical Examination

Cognitive Level: Apply

16. Type B

There are three primary tympanogram types. Type A is normal; type B reveals no mobility, typically associated with an effusion or perforation; and type C demonstrates a retracted TM, classically associated with eustachian tube dysfunction.

Blueprint Task: Using Diagnostic and Laboratory Studies

Cognitive Level: Apply

17. 6 months of age

Blueprint Task: Health Maintenance, Patient Education, and Preventive Measures

Cognitive Level: Recall

18. Acetazolamide

The clinical vignette supports the diagnosis of acute closure glaucoma. The shadowing on the iris represents the abnormal finding of a crescent shadow due to increased intraocular pressure.

Blueprint Task: Pharmaceutical Therapeutics

Cognitive Level: Apply

19. Pterygium

A pterygium may slowly grow from the nasal side across the cornea and can compromise vision.

Blueprint Task: Formulating Most Likely Diagnosis

Cognitive Level: Apply

20. Intranasal corticosteroids

The clinical vignette supports the diagnosis of moderate-severe seasonal allergic rhinitis. The intranasal corticosteroid is the optimal recommendation for this patient due to efficacy and her preference to avoid oral medications.

Blueprint Task: Clinical Intervention

Cognitive Level: Apply

21. Kiesselbach's plexus

Blueprint Task: Applying Basic Scientific Concepts

Cognitive Level: Recall

22. Soft-tissue lateral neck x-ray

Diagnosis of retropharyngeal abscess or cellulitis is supported by radiographic finding of widening of the retropharyngeal space at C2. Additional imaging such as CT may be utilized based on the patient's condition. If signs of airway compromise, airway management is critical prior to imaging.

Blueprint Task: Using Diagnostic and Laboratory Studies

Cognitive Level: Analyze

23. A 52-year-old man with Wilson disease is found to have a brown ring on the outer aspect of the cornea. What is this ocular finding?

24. A 60-year-old man with a history of constipation presents to the emergency department with a bright localized area of redness on the medial aspect of the left eye. He denies eye pain, discharge, trauma, bleeding tendencies, or problems with vision. The physical exam is normal except for the findings shown in the following photo. What is the most appropriate patient education in the management of the presumptive diagnosis?

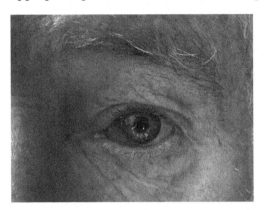

25. A 40-year-old woman presents to the emergency department with painful progressive unilateral vision loss over the past 48 hours. She describes experiencing flashing lights in her field of vision. Physical exam reveals increased pain with extraocular movement and no abnormalities to the optic nerve on fundoscopy. What is the most likely diagnosis?

26. A 44-year-old woman presents to the clinic with vertigo when she rolls over in bed or ties her shoes. The vertigo is transient, lasting a few seconds to a minute. What repositioning maneuver may alleviate her symptoms?

27. A 20-year-old baseball player sustained blunt trauma to the right eye after being struck by a ball. He is experiencing photophobia, vision loss, and pain. Inspection of the eye reveals blood in the anterior chamber without signs of an open globe injury. Extraocular movements are intact with normal upward gaze. What diagnostic test is utilized to confirm the most likely diagnosis and allows for serial monitoring?

28. A 28-year-old man presents to the clinic with an acutely tender, swollen, focal red area to the upper eyelid that is unresponsive to warm compresses. What pharmacological therapy is recommended during the acute stage?

29. What organism causes the majority of cases of malignant otitis externa?

30. A 63-year-old man with a history of brain neoplasm presents to the clinic with increasing headaches and nausea over the last 48 hours. Visual acuity is normal. Fundoscopic exam reveals papilledema. What does this ophthalmologic finding represent?

(See answers next page.)

23. Kayser–Fleischer ring

Wilson disease leads to copper accumulation in multiple organs such as the liver and brain. Kayser–Fleisher rings represent the deposition of copper in the cornea.

Blueprint Task: History Taking and Performing Physical Examination

Cognitive Level: Apply

24. Reassure and observe

The clinical vignette supports the diagnosis of subconjunctival hemorrhage, which is typically self-limited. Constipation with straining during defecation may have contributed to the hemorrhage.

Blueprint Task: Health Maintenance, Patient Education, and Preventive Measures

Cognitive Level: Analyze

25. Optic neuritis

The clinical vignette describes a classic ocular presentation of multiple sclerosis. The optic nerve often appears normal but may reveal disc edema.

Blueprint Task: Formulating Most Likely Diagnosis

Cognitive Level: Apply

26. Epley maneuver

The clinical vignette supports the diagnosis of benign paroxysmal positional vertigo.

Blueprint Task: Clinical Intervention

Cognitive Level: Apply

27. Measurement of the intraocular pressure (IOP)

The clinical vignette supports the diagnosis of traumatic hyphema. Urgent measurement of the IOP is recommended to guide management and prevent permanent vision loss. IOPs should be completed with caution by an ophthalmologist.

Blueprint Task: Using Diagnostic and Laboratory Studies

Cognitive Level: Analyze

28. Bacitracin or erythromycin ointment

The clinical vignette supports the diagnosis of hordeolum. Ophthalmologist may utilize an antibiotic/glucocorticoid combination.

Blueprint Task: Pharmaceutical Therapeutics

Cognitive Level: Analyze

29. *Pseudomonas aeruginosa*

Blueprint Task: Applying Basic Scientific Concepts

Cognitive Level: Recall

30. Increased intracranial pressure

Typical findings indicative of papilledema include blurred disc margins and optic disc swelling.

Blueprint Task: History Taking and Performing Physical Examination

Cognitive Level: Apply

31. A 24-year-old man with asthma presents to the clinic with a 3-day history of thick, white plaques on the buccal mucosa and tongue. On physical exam, the white plaques brush away with a tongue blade, but the tissue beneath is inflamed. The patient was started on an inhaled corticosteroid two months ago. What patient education is important regarding the use of an inhaled corticosteroid to prevent recurrence of the presumptive diagnosis?

32. A 2-year-old boy presents to the emergency department with fever, cough, hoarseness, and difficulty breathing. His mother describes the cough as a "barking seal." Physical exam reveals inspiratory stridor and chest retractions. Neck radiograph demonstrates a narrowed trachea and subglottis. What two pharmacologic therapies are most appropriate for the presumptive diagnosis?

33. A 45-year-old man presents to the clinic with right-sided hearing loss following years of loud noise exposure in his work environment. There is no visible abnormality on examination of the ear. Weber test lateralizes to the left, and Rinne test reveals air conduction greater than bone conduction on the right. What type of hearing loss is most likely?

34. A patient with recent ethmoid sinusitis presents to the clinic with fever, left eye pain that increases with eye movement, and decreased visual acuity. Physical exam reveals periorbital swelling and erythema, mild proptosis, and abnormal pupillary response. What diagnostic study is definitive for the most likely diagnosis?

35. A 74-year-old man presents to the emergency department with acute onset of unilateral swelling along the right angle of the jaw. He is febrile with decreased skin turgor and dry mucous membranes. Pus can be expressed from the Stensen's duct. What is the preferred pharmacologic treatment for the presumptive diagnosis?

36. What is the most common class of medication that increases the risk of cataract development?

37. An 11-year-old soccer player presents to the clinic with a 5-day history of sore throat, fever, and fatigue. Evaluation reveals exudative tonsillitis and a positive heterophile antibody. He requests to return to soccer tomorrow after resting. When is the earliest this patient can return to play, given the presumptive diagnosis?

(See answers next page.)

31. Rinse the mouth after each dose

The clinical vignette supports the diagnosis of oral candidiasis (thrush) and is treated with an antifungal.

Blueprint Task: Health Maintenance, Patient Education, and Preventive Measures

Cognitive Level: Apply

32. Steroids and nebulized racemic epinephrine

The clinical vignette supports the diagnosis of laryngotracheobronchitis, also known as croup. Both steroids and nebulized racemic epinephrine are recommended in this patient due to severity of presentation.

Blueprint Task: Clinical Intervention

Cognitive Level: Analyze

33. Right sensorineural

The exposure to loud volumes may have led to inner ear or cochlear nerve damage. In sensorineural hearing loss, the Weber test lateralizes to the unaffected side and the Rinne test reveals air conduction greater than bone conduction on the affected side.

Blueprint Task: Formulating Most Likely Diagnosis

Cognitive Level: Analyze

34. CT scan of left orbit

The clinical vignette supports the diagnosis of orbital cellulitis, which is an emergent condition. CT scan of orbit with contrast differentiates preseptal from orbital cellulitis and evaluates the extent of tissue involvement.

Blueprint Task: Using Diagnostic and Laboratory Studies

Cognitive Level: Analyze

35. Empiric antibiotic therapy

The clinical vignette supports the diagnosis of suppurative parotitis. First-line antibiotics should provide coverage for *staphylococcal* and *streptococcal* species. Additional interventions including culture and imaging may be necessary.

Blueprint Task: Pharmaceutical Therapeutics

Cognitive Level: Apply

36. Corticosteroids

Blueprint Task: Applying Basic Scientific Concepts

Cognitive Level: Recall

37. Four weeks

The clinical vignette supports the diagnosis of mononucleosis. Even if the clinical exam reveals no palpable splenomegaly, there is still a risk for splenic rupture. If splenomegaly is present, return to sports may be further delayed.

Blueprint Task: Health Maintenance, Patient Education, and Preventive Measures

Cognitive Level: Analyze

38. A 28-year-old man presents to the clinic with left eye pain, photophobia, increased lacrimation, and foreign body sensation that began while mowing the lawn 2 hours ago. He denies any known chemical exposure or contact lens use. Eye exam reveals equal and reactive pupils, normal visual acuity, and no foreign body with lid eversion. What is the most appropriate next step in the evaluation of this patient?

39. What term describes outward displacement of the lid margin?

40. A 16-year-old patient presents to the clinic with a progressively worsening sore throat, primarily on the right, fever of 38.9°C (102°F), and dysphagia. Physical exam reveals slightly muffled voice and marked erythema of the right anterior tonsillar pillar with deviation of the uvula. What is the most likely diagnosis?

41. A 3-year-old unvaccinated girl presents with acute fever, sore throat, drooling, stridor, and respiratory distress. Lateral neck radiograph demonstrates an enlarged epiglottis or "thumbprint" sign. What vaccination might have prevented the presumptive diagnosis?

42. A 21-year-old man with no medical problems presents with rapid, painless, monocular vision loss. Fundoscopic exam reveals retinal hemorrhages along with optic disc edema, demonstrating a "blood and thunder" appearance. What laboratory study should be considered to determine the cause of the presumptive diagnosis?

43. A 74-year-old man with type 2 diabetes and coronary artery disease presents to the clinic with right-sided ptosis. An abnormality of which cranial nerve is most likely causing the ptosis?

44. In addition to topical antibiotics and maintaining a dry ear canal, what clinical intervention is recommended in the treatment of an acquired cholesteatoma?

45. A 34-year-old woman with long-standing allergic rhinitis presents to the clinic with nasal congestion, rhinorrhea, and sneezing since discontinuing her allergy medication one year ago. Physical exam reveals bilateral painless pale growths on the nasal mucosa. What do these growths most likely represent?

(*See answers next page.*)

38. Fluorescein stain
Fluorescein stain is helpful to identify corneal epithelial defects occurring in conditions such as corneal abrasion or injury.
Blueprint Task: Clinical Intervention
Cognitive Level: Apply

39. Ectropion
Blueprint Task: History Taking and Performing Physical Examination
Cognitive Level: Recall

40. Right tonsillar abscess
"Hot potato voice" describes the muffled voice characteristically seen in patients with tonsillar abscess. Typical treatment includes drainage and empiric antibiotics.
Blueprint Task: Formulating Most Likely Diagnosis
Cognitive Level: Analyze

41. Haemophilus influenzae type B vaccine
The clinical vignette supports the diagnosis of epiglottis, a potentially life-threatening condition, commonly caused by *Haemophilus influenzae B*.
Blueprint Task: Health Maintenance, Patient Education, and Preventive Measures
Cognitive Level: Analyze

42. Thrombophilia screen
The clinical vignette supports the diagnosis of central retinal vascular occlusion (CRVO). In a young patient with CRVO, coagulopathy must be considered as a source for thrombi.
Blueprint Task: Using Diagnostic and Laboratory Studies
Cognitive Level: Analyze

43. Cranial nerve III (oculomotor nerve)
Blueprint Task: Applying Basic Scientific Concepts
Cognitive Level: Recall

44. Debridement
These clinical interventions reduce inflammation and prevent infection.
Blueprint Task: Clinical Intervention
Cognitive Level: Apply

45. Nasal polyps
Nasal polyps can result from chronic inflammation common in conditions such as recurrent sinusitis and allergic rhinitis. Intranasal corticosteroids are commonly used as initial therapy for nasal polyps.
Blueprint Task: History Taking and Performing Physical Examination
Cognitive Level: Apply

46. An 8-year-old girl, with incomplete immunization status, presents to the clinic with 2-day history of cough, rhinorrhea, sore throat, and fever. Physical exam reveals small white specks on the buccal mucosa by the second molars. There is no skin rash. What is the most likely diagnosis?

47. A 25-year-old man presents with left ear pain and fullness that began on a scuba diving trip. Physical exam reveals conductive hearing loss and hemotympanum of the left ear. What is the most appropriate pharmacologic treatment for the presumptive diagnosis?

48. Chronic elevation in uric acid may lead to monosodium urate crystal deposits on the helix or antihelix of the ears. What term describes these firm nodules associated with gout?

49. A 35-year-old woman presents to the clinic with fever and pain behind the left ear. Symptoms have progressively worsened over the past few weeks following ineffective treatment of left acute otitis media. Physical exam reveals postauricular erythema and tenderness. What imaging study is recommended to evaluate for the presumptive diagnosis?

50. A 33-year-old woman describes recurrent "ringing, whooshing, and buzzing" sounds in the absence of hearing loss. What diagnostic study is recommended to evaluate for the presumptive diagnosis?

51. A 22-year-old man with neurofibromatosis type 2 (NF2) presents to the clinic with unilateral sensorineural hearing loss, tinnitus, and gait imbalance. MRI reveals an abnormal lesion in the internal auditory canal. What is the presumptive diagnosis?

52. Conditions such as malignant otitis externa and tonsillar abscess may cause spasm of the jaw muscles. What term describes these spasms?

53. A 32-year-old woman presents to the clinic with progressively worsening nasal congestion, yellow-green nasal discharge, facial pressure, dental pain, and a fever of 39.1°C (102.3°F). What two organisms are most commonly associated with the presumptive diagnosis?

(See answers next page.)

46. Measles
Koplik spots are the classic enanthem strongly associated with measles (rubeola). The associated skin rash is often not visible until symptoms have been present for 3–5 days.
Blueprint Task: Formulating Most Likely Diagnosis
Cognitive Level: Analyze

47. Oral decongestants
The clinical vignette supports the diagnosis of barotitis secondary to barotrauma of descent.
Blueprint Task: Pharmaceutical Therapeutics
Cognitive Level: Analyze

48. Tophi
Blueprint Task: History Taking and Performing Physical Examination
Cognitive Level: Recall

49. CT scan of head
The clinical vignette supports the diagnosis of mastoiditis. CT classically demonstrates coalescence of mastoid air cells.
Blueprint Task: Using Diagnostic and Laboratory Studies
Cognitive Level: Analyze

50. Audiometry
The clinical vignette supports the diagnosis of non-pulsatile tinnitus without hearing loss. Audiometry would be normal. Patient education should include avoidance of ototoxic agents, limiting exposure to excessive noise, and incorporating music to mask the sound.
Blueprint Task: Clinical Intervention
Cognitive Level: Analyze

51. Vestibular schwannoma
Vestibular schwannomas (also known as "acoustic neuromas") are tumors that develop from the vestibulocochlear (VIII) cranial nerve. These tumors are more common in patients with NF2.
Blueprint Task: Formulating Most Likely Diagnosis
Cognitive Level: Apply

52. Trismus
Blueprint Task: History Taking and Performing Physical Examination
Cognitive Level: Recall

53. *S. Pneumoniae, H. influenza*
The clinical vignette supports the diagnosis of acute bacterial sinusitis. Less common organisms include *Staphylococcus aureus* and *Moraxella catarrhalis*. Viral etiology is unlikely due to severity of symptoms.
Blueprint Task: Applying Basic Scientific Concepts
Cognitive Level: Analyze

54. A 35-year-old woman presents to the clinic with vertigo, nausea, unilateral hearing loss, and tinnitus over the past 3 days. History reveals a recent upper respiratory infection. She is currently taking an anti-emetic. What initial class of medication may be recommended to provide symptomatic relief?

55. What ocular condition is commonly associated with a history of atopy and the presence of chemosis?

56. A 62-year-old man presents to the clinic with an acute right-sided vision loss. He denies pain or ocular discharge. Physical exam reveals complete vision loss with no light perception in the right eye (OD) and the left eye (OS) is 20/20. There is an afferent pupillary defect in the right eye. On fundoscopic exam, the retina appears whitened with a cherry-red spot. What is the most likely diagnosis?

57. A 34-year-old man presents to the clinic with a 2-day history of left ear pain, pruritus, and discharge. He went scuba diving a week ago. On physical exam, the left tragus and pinna are tender upon manipulation, and there is erythema and edema of the ear canal with purulent discharge. What treatment is most appropriate for the presumptive diagnosis?

58. A 35-year-old woman presents to the clinic with acute on chronic "canker sores." Examination of the oral mucosa reveals a few small, shallow, tender, erythematous ulcers. In addition to oral hygiene and avoidance of triggers, what is the first-line pharmacologic therapy to provide symptomatic relief for the presumptive diagnosis?

59. What condition is characteristically associated with episodic vertigo, hearing loss, tinnitus, and ear fullness?

60. A 62-year-old man recently completed multiple rounds of antibiotics. He presents to the clinic with recent development of dark tongue discoloration and bad taste in the mouth. What is the cause of the tongue discoloration?

61. A 2-year-old patient presents to the clinic to establish care with a well-child examination. Physical exam reveals an abnormal corneal light reflection and an abnormal cover-uncover test. What is the most appropriate next step given the presumptive diagnosis?

(See answers next page.)

54. Antihistamine
The clinical vignette supports a diagnosis of vestibular labyrinthitis. Meclizine is a commonly utilized medication.
Blueprint Task: *Pharmaceutical Therapeutics*
Cognitive Level: *Apply*

55. Allergic conjunctivitis
Blueprint Task: *History Taking and Performing Physical Examination*
Cognitive Level: *Recall*

56. Central retinal artery occlusion (CRAO)
In a patient with CRAO, there is obstruction of blood flow to the retina, which results in a pale appearance. The blood supply to the macula is unobstructed, leading to the cherry-red spot.
Blueprint Task: *Formulating Most Likely Diagnosis*
Cognitive Level: *Apply*

57. Otic antibiotic
The clinical vignette supports the diagnosis of otitis externa. Otic antibiotics are available with or without a corticosteroid. Options include aminoglycoside (neomycin/polymyxin B) or fluoroquinolone (ciprofloxacin). If tympanic membrane perforation cannot be ruled out, aminoglycosides are to be avoided due to potential ototoxicity.
Blueprint Task: *Clinical Intervention*
Cognitive Level: *Analyze*

58. Topical corticosteroids
The clinical vignette supports the diagnosis of recurrent aphthous stomatitis. Topical corticosteroids are the primary treatment; however, topical anesthetics may also be beneficial.
Blueprint Task: *Pharmaceutical Therapeutics*
Cognitive Level: *Analyze*

59. Ménière's disease
Blueprint Task: *History Taking and Performing Physical Examination*
Cognitive Level: *Recall*

60. Elongated filiform papillae
The clinical vignette supports the diagnosis of black hairy tongue. This condition increases with antibiotic and tobacco use.
Blueprint Task: *Formulating Most Likely Diagnosis*
Cognitive Level: *Apply*

61. Refer to ophthalmology
The clinical vignette supports the diagnosis of strabismus. The corneal light reflection and cover-uncover test are abnormal due to ocular misalignment. Early referral to ophthalmology, with assessment of visual acuity, is necessary to decrease the risk of amblyopia.
Blueprint Task: *Clinical Intervention*
Cognitive Level: *Analyze*

62. A 27-year-old professional singer presents with hoarseness and is diagnosed with laryngitis. In addition to educating the patient to avoid vigorous use of her voice, what class of medication may be considered, given her career, to help speed recovery?

63. A 78-year-old man with hypertension, poorly fitting dentures, and a history of nutritional deficiencies is found to have inflammation, soreness, and fissuring at the corners of the mouth. What vitamin is most likely deficient?

64. A 45-year-old man presents to the emergency department with fever and worsening left eye pain and edema over the past 24 hours. Physical exam reveals periorbital swelling with erythema, proptosis, and painful restricted extraocular movements. Based on the presumptive diagnosis, what treatment is recommended?

65. A 63-year-old woman presents to the clinic with left eye pain and redness since this morning. The patient wears contact lenses for several consecutive days. Physical exam reveals mild visual acuity loss in the left eye with a white infiltrate noted on penlight exam. What is the most likely diagnosis?

66. A 21-year-old woman presents to the clinic with swelling and pruritis of the upper lip that occurred after eating shellfish. She does not have any dysphagia, difficulty breathing, rash, or gastrointestinal symptoms. What term describes the localized swelling of the lip?

(*See answers next page.*)

62. Corticosteroids

For typical laryngitis, steroids are not needed; however, as the hoarseness is affecting her occupation, more aggressive management is necessary. If hoarseness does not resolve with conservative therapy, a referral to otolaryngology for laryngoscope is recommended.

Blueprint Task: *Pharmaceutical Therapeutics*

Cognitive Level: *Apply*

63. Vitamin B

The clinical vignette supports the diagnosis of angular cheilitis. Additional risks include factors such as dentures and advanced age.

Blueprint Task: *History Taking and Performing Physical Examination*

Cognitive Level: *Analyze*

64. Empiric antibiotic therapy

The clinical vignette supports the diagnosis of orbital cellulitis. Immediate administration of intravenous antibiotics is recommended to prevent extension of infection and optic nerve damage.

Blueprint Task: *Pharmaceutical Therapeutics*

Cognitive Level: *Analyze*

65. Corneal ulcer

Contact lens overuse can result in corneal ulceration and hypopyon.

Blueprint Task: *Formulating Most Likely Diagnosis*

Cognitive Level: *Apply*

66. Angioedema

Angioedema, commonly caused by an allergic reaction, may lead to progressive airway obstruction if the throat or tongue is involved.

Blueprint Task: *Formulating Most Likely Diagnosis*

Cognitive Level: *Apply*

Gastrointestinal System/Nutrition

1. What condition is associated with Charcot's triad defined by right upper quadrant pain, jaundice, and fever?

2. A 54-year-old man with type 2 diabetes and a recent HbA1c of 12.4% presents to the clinic with upper abdominal pain, early satiety, nausea, and vomiting 1–3 hours after meals. What imaging study is most helpful in the evaluation of the presumptive diagnosis?

3. A 42-year-old man with a history of cholelithiasis presents to the emergency department with fever, tachycardia, and upper abdominal pain that radiates straight through to his back. The pain is worse lying supine and improved sitting up and leaning forward. On physical exam, the abdomen is tender in the epigastric region with no guarding or rebound tenderness. Lipase is greater than three times the upper normal limit. What scoring criteria are helpful in assessing the severity of the presumptive diagnosis?

4. A 45-year-old man presents with a 2-day history of fever, pain with defecation, and rectal discharge. On physical exam, a tender, fluctuant mass is palpated in the midline posterior aspect of the rectal canal. What is the appropriate treatment?

5. A 57-year-old man with osteoarthritis presents to the clinic with a 2-month history of epigastric abdominal pain. The pain is described as burning, gnawing, and is aggravated by meals. Symptoms occur within 30 minutes of meal ingestion. Famotidine has provided only partial relief. What class of medication is most commonly the cause of the presumptive diagnosis?

6. What nutrient deficiency is common in patients with chronic alcohol use and can be associated with beriberi or Wernicke–Korsakoff syndrome?

7. A 70-year-old man presents to the clinic with progressive jaundice, right upper quadrant abdominal pain, and unintentional weight loss. Previous ultrasounds demonstrate gallbladder polyps >1 cm and calcification of the gallbladder. What is the most likely diagnosis?

8. What condition results in loss of synthetic function of the liver leading to thrombocytopenia, prolonged prothrombin time, increased INR, and hypoalbuminemia?

1. Ascending cholangitis
Blueprint Task: History Taking and Performing Physical Examination
Cognitive Level: Recall

2. Gastric emptying scan
The clinical vignette supports the diagnosis of gastroparesis characterized by delayed gastric emptying associated with autonomic neuropathy. Poorly controlled diabetes increases the risk. A gastric emptying scan helps assess the rate of solid food emptying over interval time periods.
Blueprint Task: Using Diagnostic and Laboratory Studies
Cognitive Level: Analyze

3. Ranson criteria
The clinical vignette supports the diagnosis of acute pancreatitis. The Ranson criteria are utilized to predict the course, prognosis, and mortality rate associated with the diagnosis. Two common etiologies for the development of pancreatitis include cholelithiasis and alcohol use.
Blueprint Task: Formulating Most Likely Diagnosis
Cognitive Level: Analyze

4. Surgical drainage
The clinical vignette is indicative of an intersphincteric (perirectal) abscess, which should be referred to a surgeon to be drained.
Blueprint Task: Clinical Intervention
Cognitive Level: Analyze

5. NSAIDs
The clinical vignette supports the diagnosis of a gastric ulcer. Concomitant use of other medications such as corticosteroids and anticoagulants may complicate peptic ulcer disease.
Blueprint Task: Pharmaceutical Therapeutics
Cognitive Level: Analyze

6. Thiamine
Blueprint Task: Applying Basic Scientific Concepts
Cognitive Level: Recall

7. Carcinoma of the gallbladder
The clinical vignette and ultrasound finding of gallbladder calcification (porcelain gallbladder) supports gallbladder cancer.
Blueprint Task: Formulating Most Likely Diagnosis
Cognitive Level: Apply

8. Cirrhosis
Blueprint Task: Using Diagnostic and Laboratory Studies
Cognitive Level: Recall

9. During a specialized physical exam, the clinician places a hand just above the right knee and asks the patient to raise the thigh against resistance while laying supine. Increased pain in the right lower quadrant represents what sign?

10. A 48-year-old woman with no chronic medical conditions presents with a 24-hour history of fever, bloody diarrhea with frequent small stools, tenesmus, and abdominal pain with cramping. She returned from a trip abroad 2 days ago. What primary treatment is recommended while awaiting stool culture?

11. A 67-year-old woman with gastroparesis continues to experience early satiety, postprandial nausea and vomiting, and epigastric discomfort despite small frequent low-fat meals. What medication can assist with motility but also may be associated with tardive dyskinesia?

12. What gram-negative organism has been implicated in the development of peptic ulcer disease and gastric cancer?

13. A 24-year-old man is brought into the emergency department 2 hours after ingesting half of a bottle of aspirin. The patient's airway, breathing, and circulation are stable. He received aggressive fluid replacement and activated charcoal. Metabolic abnormalities are being monitored. What additional treatment is beneficial in reducing salicylate toxicity?

14. A 30-year-old man presents to the emergency department with dysphagia and a food impaction. An esophagogastroduodenoscopy (EGD) reveals concentric rings and strictures. What condition is commonly associated with this diagnosis?

15. A 72-year-old man with chronic constipation presents to the emergency department with progressively worsening abdominal pain, vomiting, and obstipation over the last 48 hours. Plain abdominal radiograph reveals a dilated sigmoid colon. What is the most likely diagnosis?

16. What nutrient deficiency presents with macrocytic anemia and can be associated with peripheral neuropathy?

(See answers next page.)

9. Psoas sign
The psoas sign may indicate conditions such as appendicitis, peritonitis, and psoas abscess.
Blueprint Task: History Taking and Performing Physical Examination
Cognitive Level: Apply

10. Empiric antibiotic
The clinical vignette suggests an acute, inflammatory diarrhea with characteristics of *Shigella*. Ceftriaxone, levofloxacin, or ciprofloxacin are the most commonly utilized antibiotics.
Blueprint Task: Clinical Intervention
Cognitive Level: Analyze

11. Metoclopramide
Tardive dyskinesia is a medication-induced movement disorder causing repetitive, involuntary movements such as grimacing, lip smacking, and tongue protrusion.
Blueprint Task: Pharmaceutical Therapeutics
Cognitive Level: Apply

12. *Helicobacter pylori*
Blueprint Task: Applying Basic Scientific Concepts
Cognitive Level: Recall

13. Systemic and urinary alkalization
Along with volume resuscitation with either normal saline or lactated Ringers, patients with moderate to severe salicylate overdose should also be treated with bicarbonate to maintain serum and urinary pH around 7.5.
Blueprint Task: Clinical Intervention
Cognitive Level: Analyze

14. Atopy
The clinical vignette supports the diagnosis of eosinophilic esophagitis, which is more commonly found in individuals with a history of atopy. Atopy includes asthma, atopic dermatitis, allergic rhinitis, and food allergies.
Blueprint Task: History Taking and Performing Physical Examination
Cognitive Level: Analyze

15. Sigmoid volvulus
Risk factors include conditions such as chronic constipation and/or redundant sigmoid colon.
Blueprint Task: Formulating Most Likely Diagnosis
Cognitive Level: Apply

16. Vitamin B12
Blueprint Task: Applying Basic Scientific Concepts
Cognitive Level: Recall

17. A 54-year-old man with cirrhosis and ascites has been unresponsive to dietary salt restrictions. What class of medication may be initiated to help manage his ascites?

18. Antimicrobial therapy is avoided in patients with *E. coli 0157:H7* as it may increase the risk of what condition?

19. What medication used for obesity management commonly causes distressing gastrointestinal side effects, which should be disclosed prior to starting the medication?

20. A patient presents to the emergency department approximately 20 hours after onset of a thrombosed external hemorrhoid. What definitive procedure would be recommended?

21. A 21-year-old woman with type 1 diabetes presents with a 6-month history of diarrhea, bloating, flatulence, and weight loss. Labs reveal a normal total IgA level, elevated tissue transglutaminase IgA, and positive endomysial antibody. What dermatologic condition is associated with the presumptive diagnosis?

22. A 56-year-old man with a history of HIV and anal condylomas presents to the clinic with anorectal pain and an annular lesion. What is the most likely diagnosis?

23. A 67-year-old man with a 30-pack-year smoking history is advised to have an abdominal ultrasound to screen for what condition?

24. A 57-year-old man with diabetes mellitus and chronic pancreatitis develops weight loss and steatorrhea. Laboratory evaluation reveals elevated fecal fat and decreased fecal elastase level. What pharmacologic therapy is recommended for the presumptive diagnosis?

25. What condition is associated with inflammatory bowel disease (IBD) and can lead to fatigue, pruritus, jaundice, and a cholestatic liver pattern?

(*See answers next page.*)

17. Diuretics

The two most commonly utilized diuretics, used independently or in combination, are spironolactone and furosemide.

Blueprint Task: *Pharmaceutical Therapeutics*
Cognitive Level: *Apply*

18. Hemolytic uremic syndrome

Blueprint Task: *Clinical Intervention*
Cognitive Level: *Recall*

19. Orlistat

Side effects of orlistat include the reduction in absorption of fat-soluble vitamins, abdominal discomfort, flatulence with oily discharge, and fecal urgency.

Blueprint Task: *Health Maintenance, Patient Education, and Preventive Measures*
Cognitive Level: *Apply*

20. Excision

Blueprint Task: *Clinical Intervention*
Cognitive Level: *Recall*

21. Dermatitis herpetiformis

The clinical vignette supports the diagnosis of Celiac disease, an immune-mediated disorder triggered by the ingestion of gluten. It can present with intestinal and extraintestinal manifestations.

Blueprint Task: *History Taking and Performing Physical Examination*
Cognitive Level: *Analyze*

22. Anal squamous cell carcinoma

HIV and anal condylomas are risk factors for the development of anal cancer.

Blueprint Task: *Formulating Most Likely Diagnosis*
Cognitive Level: *Apply*

23. Abdominal aortic aneurysm

Blueprint Task: *Health Maintenance, Patient Education, and Preventive Measures*
Cognitive Level: *Recall*

24. Pancreatic enzyme replacement therapy (PERT)

The clinical vignette supports a diagnosis of exocrine pancreatic insufficiency, which can result in malabsorption. PERT provides lipase to aid in fat digestion.

Blueprint Task: *Pharmaceutical Therapeutics*
Cognitive Level: *Analyze*

25. Primary Sclerosing Cholangitis (PSC)

PSC is associated with IBD in ulcerative colitis more than Crohn disease. PSC can be associated with development of cholangiocarcinoma.

Blueprint Task: *Applying Basic Scientific Concepts*
Cognitive Level: *Apply*

26. A patient reports daily heartburn when lying down, as well as 30-60 minutes after a meal. Antacids and H2 blockers have been ineffective. Besides lifestyle modifications, what pharmaceutical therapy is recommended for the suspected diagnosis?

27. What class of medication may be given to patients with inflammatory bowel disease for short-term use to treat an acute flare but may lead to complications including mood changes, weight gain, elevated blood glucose, osteoporosis, and cataracts?

28. A 23-year-old woman presents to the clinic with intermittent episodes of bloating, gas, loose stools, and crampy abdominal pain following consumption of milk-containing products. What is the most likely diagnosis?

29. A 52-year-old woman presents to the emergency department with fever, nausea, vomiting, left lower quadrant abdominal pain, and diarrhea. Colonoscopy completed at age 50 revealed moderate sigmoid diverticulosis. Complete blood count reveals leukocytosis. What imaging study is most appropriate given the presumptive diagnosis?

30. A 67-year-old woman with a history of hepatitis C and chronic alcohol use presents to the clinic with ascites and visible abdominal wall veins. These clinical features stem from what complication associated with her condition?

31. A 67-year-old man presents with epigastric abdominal pain, early satiety, decreased appetite, and weight loss. He has a history of chronic *H. pylori* infection. Physical exam reveals a left supraclavicular node and umbilical nodule. What is the presumptive diagnosis?

32. In a 71-year-old woman with a documented history of osteoporosis and high risk for falls, what laboratory test should be considered to determine the dosing of supplemental vitamin D?

33. A 55-year-old man presents to the clinic with an anal fissure. He has tried fiber supplements and sitz baths with minimal relief. What two topical therapies are recommended for the conservative management of the anal fissure?

(See answers next page.)

26. Proton pump inhibitor
The clinical vignette supports the diagnosis of gastroesophageal reflux disease (GERD).
Blueprint Task: Pharmaceutical Therapeutics
Cognitive Level: Analyze

27. Corticosteroids
Blueprint Task: Health Maintenance, Patient Education, and Preventive Measures
Cognitive Level: Recall

28. Lactose intolerance
Lactose intolerance results from a lactase deficiency. Lactase is necessary to break down lactose into glucose and galactose.
Blueprint Task: Formulating Most Likely Diagnosis
Cognitive Level: Apply

29. CT scan of abdomen and pelvis
The clinical vignette supports the diagnosis of diverticulitis. CT of abdomen and pelvis with oral and IV contrast is recommended to evaluate for evidence of diverticulitis and complications including abscess, fistula, obstruction, and perforation.
Blueprint Task: Using Diagnostic and Laboratory Studies
Cognitive Level: Analyze

30. Portal hypertension
Clinical manifestations of portal hypertension, a complication of cirrhosis, includes ascites, splenomegaly, caput medusae, esophageal and rectal varices, and hepatic encephalopathy. Cirrhosis is characterized by scarring, fibrosis, and nodularity of the liver, which can lead to increase pressure within the portal venous system.
Blueprint Task: Applying Basic Scientific Concepts
Cognitive Level: Analyze

31. Metastatic gastric adenocarcinoma
The clinical vignette and evidence of Virchow node and Sister Mary Joseph nodule, respectively, suggest gastric adenocarcinoma.
Blueprint Task: History Taking and Performing Physical Examination
Cognitive Level: Apply

32. 25-OH vitamin D level
Blueprint Task: Health Maintenance, Patient Education, and Preventive Measures
Cognitive Level: Recall

33. Anesthetics and vasodilators
Anesthetics relieve pain while vasodilators relax the anal sphincter and promote healing. If constipation is present, additional patient education is warranted.
Blueprint Task: Clinical Intervention
Cognitive Level: Apply

34. Most colorectal cancers arise from what type of colon polyps?

35. A 32-year-old woman with terminal ileum Crohn disease is initiated on methotrexate therapy. Which nutrient is necessary to supplement while on this therapy?

36. A 45-year-old man reports bone pain in his right thigh and pelvis that is worse at night. Labs reveal a significantly elevated alkaline phosphatase. Radiographs reveal "flame-shaped" lesions in the right femur. What is the preferred medication for the presumptive diagnosis?

37. A 55-year-old man with diabetes mellitus is found to have abnormal labs, including elevated aspartate aminotransferase, alkaline phosphatase, serum iron, and ferritin. On physical exam, the skin reveals bronze pigmentation. Serum cortisol level is normal. The patient was encouraged to avoid iron-rich foods. What clinical intervention may be considered based on the presumptive diagnosis?

38. An 18-year-old woman presents to the clinic with a 1-week history of malaise, anorexia, nausea, and vomiting. She returned from a summer trip abroad in Asia one month ago. Physical exam reveals, temperature of 38.0°C (100.4°F), jaundice, right upper quadrant tenderness, and hepatomegaly. Follow-up labs reveal AST/ALT >1000 mg/dL, Hep A IgM (+), Hep Bs Ag (−), Hep Bc IgM (−), Hep C Ab (−). What is the presumptive diagnosis?

39. What imaging study may precipitate toxic megacolon in a patient with severe ulcerative colitis?

40. A 65-year-old man presents to the clinic with a 2 to 3-day history of foul-smelling, watery diarrhea, and abdominal cramps. He completed a course of clindamycin a few days ago for a dental infection, and 2 weeks prior was treated inpatient for a complicated course of diverticulitis. What two primary risk factors in this patient increase the suspicion for the presumptive diagnosis?

41. When should a proton pump inhibitor (PPI) be taken in relation to meals?

42. A 4-week-old boy presents with projectile vomiting that is nonbilious in nature. On physical exam, an olive-shaped mass is palpated in the epigastrium. What is the definitive treatment for the presumptive diagnosis?

(See answers next page.)

34. Adenomas

Adenomas are precancerous colon polyps and include tubular, tubulovillous, and villous. The adenoma to carcinoma sequence is approximately 10 years. Other types of colon polyps include sessile serrated, hyperplastic, and inflammatory pseudopolyps.

Blueprint Task: *Applying Basic Scientific Concepts*
Cognitive Level: *Apply*

35. Folate

Blueprint Task: *Pharmaceutical Therapeutics*
Cognitive Level: *Recall*

36. Zoledronic acid

The clinical vignette supports the diagnosis of Paget disease. Zoledronic acid aids in normalizing alkaline phosphatase and is the first-line treatment.

Blueprint Task: *Pharmaceutical Therapeutics*
Cognitive Level: *Analyze*

37. Therapeutic phlebotomy

The clinical vignette supports the diagnosis of hemochromatosis.

Blueprint Task: *Clinical Intervention*
Cognitive Level: *Analyze*

38. Acute hepatitis A virus (HAV) infection

The clinical presentation, incubation period, and laboratory results support the diagnosis of HAV.

Blueprint Task: *Formulating Most Likely Diagnosis*
Cognitive Level: *Analyze*

39. Barium enema

Blueprint Task: *Using Diagnostic and Laboratory Studies*
Cognitive Level: *Recall*

40. Antibiotic use and hospitalization

The clinical vignette supports the diagnosis of *Clostridioides difficile* infection.

Blueprint Task: *History Taking and Performing Physical Examination*
Cognitive Level: *Analyze*

41. 30 minutes prior to the first meal of the day

Blueprint Task: *Health Maintenance, Patient Education, and Preventive Measures*
Cognitive Level: *Recall*

42. Surgical pyloromyotomy

The clinical vignette supports the diagnosis of pyloric stenosis, which can be confirmed with ultrasonography. Clinically, the olive-shaped mass is rarely palpable.

Blueprint Task: *Clinical Intervention*
Cognitive Level: *Analyze*

43. A 47-year-old woman with chronic pain syndrome taking an opioid presents to the emergency department with vomiting, constipation, and diffuse abdominal pain. Physical exam reveals a distended abdomen with hypoactive bowel sounds. A follow-up abdominal x-ray reveals dilated loops of bowel with gas present in both the small and large intestines. What is the most likely diagnosis?

44. A 68-year-old sedentary man with a 40-pack year tobacco history and excessive alcohol use presents with jaundice and unintentional weight loss. Physical exam reveals an epigastric mass and a non-tender palpable gallbladder. CA 19-9 is elevated. What anatomic section is most commonly involved in the presumptive diagnosis?

45. What two antibiotics are first-line options in the treatment of *Clostridioides difficile* (*C. diff*) infection in the outpatient setting?

46. A 24-year-old woman presents with mild epigastric abdominal pain for the past week in the absence of other related symptoms. She admits to ingesting her own hair on a daily basis for at least 6 months. Based on her history, what is the appropriate intervention for the presumptive diagnosis?

47. A 55-year-old man with a history of alcohol use, hepatitis C, and cirrhosis should be screened for hepatocellular cancer every 6 months with what imaging and laboratory study?

48. A 42-year-old woman presents to the clinic with hunger-like epigastric abdominal pain and dyspepsia. She reports that her pain improves within 2–4 hours of meal intake. She is without hematemesis or melena. What is the presumptive diagnosis?

49. A healthy 22-year-old man presents to the clinic with intermittent jaundice. He reports a history of similar intermittent jaundice in other healthy family members. Given the most likely diagnosis, what would be the expected laboratory finding?

50. A 48-year-old man with cirrhosis presents with abdominal pain and a 10-pound weight gain over the past 2 weeks. On physical exam, the abdomen is protuberant with bulging flanks and evidence of shifting dullness. This patient is presenting with what complication associated with cirrhosis?

(See answers next page.)

43. Ileus
The clinical presentation and x-ray findings support the diagnosis of ileus likely secondary to use of hypomotility agents such as opioids.
Blueprint Task: Formulating Most Likely Diagnosis
Cognitive Level: Apply

44. Head of the pancreas
The clinical vignette supports the diagnosis of pancreatic cancer. The non-tender palpable gallbladder describes the Courvoisier sign. Most patients present with locally advanced or metastatic disease.
Blueprint Task: Applying Basic Scientific Concepts
Cognitive Level: Analyze

45. Vancomycin and fidaxomicin
Oral vancomycin or fidaxomicin are appropriate treatments of an initial and/or recurrent infection with *C. diff* in the outpatient setting. Historically, metronidazole has been utilized for *C. diff* therapy; however, the above medications represent first-line treatment.
Blueprint Task: Pharmaceutical Therapeutics
Cognitive Level: Apply

46. Removal of trichobezoar via endoscopy
Bezoars are a hard, solid mass that can form in the stomach from various substances. Trichobezoars are composed of hair.
Blueprint Task: Clinical Intervention
Cognitive Level: Analyze

47. Ultrasonography and alpha-fetoprotein
Blueprint Task: Health Maintenance, Patient Education, and Preventive Measures
Cognitive Level: Recall

48. Duodenal ulcer
Duodenal ulcers typically improve with oral intake as opposed to gastric ulcers, which worsen with oral intake.
Blueprint Task: Formulating Most Likely Diagnosis
Cognitive Level: Apply

49. Isolated unconjugated hyperbilirubinemia
The clinical vignette supports the diagnosis of Gilbert syndrome, a benign inherited condition that results in impaired conjugation of bilirubin.
Blueprint Task: Using Diagnostic and Laboratory Studies
Cognitive Level: Analyze

50. Ascites
Ascites is the collection of fluid within the peritoneal cavity.
Blueprint Task: History Taking and Performing Physical Examination
Cognitive Level: Apply

51. A 25-year-old man who regularly uses intravenous drugs presents with sepsis of unknown origin, left upper quadrant abdominal pain, and splenic enlargement. Radiographs of the chest and abdomen show a left pleural effusion along with areas of gas within the spleen. Based on the presumptive diagnosis, what is the definitive intervention?

52. A 51-year-old man with a history of erosive esophagitis has recently undergone dilation for peptic strictures. What class of medication should be considered to prevent recurrence?

53. A 51-year-old healthy woman presents for an evaluation of chronic constipation. A colonoscopy completed six months ago was unremarkable. She denies the use of hypomotility agents. Physical exam is negative for pelvic floor dysfunction, rectal prolapse, or rectocele. Laboratory workup is negative for hypercalcemia and hypothyroidism. What patient education is most important to discuss?

54. A 9-month-old presents to the emergency department with sudden onset of colicky abdominal pain and bloody mucoid stools. The mother describes inconsolable crying with the infant drawing the legs up to the abdomen. On physical exam, a sausage-shaped mass is palpated in the right upper quadrant. What is the presumptive diagnosis?

55. A patient presents with constant abdominal pain, emesis, and altered bowel function consistent with a complete small bowel obstruction. What would be the expected abnormal vital signs indicative of secondary bowel ischemia and sepsis?

56. A 54-year-old woman presents to the clinic with fatigue and pruritus. A liver panel demonstrates a cholestatic pattern. What laboratory marker would be helpful in the evaluation of the presumptive diagnosis that results in autoimmune destruction of intrahepatic bile ducts and cholestasis?

57. What is the preferred diagnostic modality to screen for esophageal varices?

58. A 2-day-old girl was found to have elevated plasma phenylalanine on her newborn screening test. The patient was diagnosed with phenylketonuria (PKU). What is the recommended clinical intervention to avoid future significant intellectual disability?

(*See answers next page.*)

51. Splenectomy

The clinical vignette supports the diagnosis of splenic abscess, which may be a potential complication from intravenous drug use. Splenectomy is recommended in stable patients.

Blueprint Task: Clinical Intervention

Cognitive Level: Analyze

52. Proton pump inhibitor

Blueprint Task: Pharmaceutical Therapeutics

Cognitive Level: Recall

53. Fiber, fluid, and exercise

The clinical vignette supports the diagnosis of chronic constipation. The history and physical exam negate the causes of constipation secondary to an obstructive process, medication, pelvic floor dysfunction, and metabolic or systemic conditions.

Blueprint Task: Health Maintenance, Patient Education, and Preventive Measures

Cognitive Level: Analyze

54. Intussusception

The classic triad of pain, bloody stools, and palpable mass suggests intussusception, although all three features may only be seen in a small number of patients.

Blueprint Task: Formulating Most Likely Diagnosis

Cognitive Level: Apply

55. Fever, hypotension, and tachycardia

Secondary bowel ischemia typically presents with fever and tachycardia. If volume depletion and sepsis are present, hypotension can manifest.

Blueprint Task: History Taking and Performing Physical Examination

Cognitive Level: Apply

56. Anti-mitochondrial antibody

The clinical vignette supports the diagnosis of primary biliary cholangitis.

Blueprint Task: Using Diagnostic and Laboratory Studies

Cognitive Level: Analyze

57. Esophagogastroduodenoscopy (EGD)

Blueprint Task: Health Maintenance, Patient Education, and Preventive Measures

Cognitive Level: Recall

58. Dietary phenylalanine restriction

PKU is caused by a reduction in the activity of phenylalanine hydroxylase. Dietary restriction should be initiated in the first weeks of life.

Blueprint Task: Clinical Intervention

Cognitive Level: Apply

59. A 60-year-old man with a history of excessive alcohol use, chronic liver disease, and secondary ascites presents with fever and abdominal pain. Paracentesis reveals neutrocytic ascites with a polymorphonuclear leukocyte (PMN) count of 500 cells/mcL. What is the most appropriate treatment for the presumptive diagnosis?

60. A 65-year-old man with a 40-pack-year tobacco history and chronic alcohol use is referred to the gastroenterologist for dysphagia and weight loss. Esophagogastroduodenoscopy (EGD) reveals a mass in the distal esophagus. Biopsy is likely to reveal which type of esophageal cancer?

61. A 48-year-old man with a 10 pack-year tobacco history and gastric ulcer presents with a sudden onset of generalized abdominal pain and a tender rigid abdomen. Follow-up imaging reveals free air under the diaphragm. What is the most likely diagnosis?

62. Once cardiac chest pain has been excluded, what historical finding would support a diagnosis of esophageal spasm as a source of chest pain?

63. A 45-year-old man with refractory peptic ulcer disease undergoes an esophagogastroduodenoscopy which reveals multiple duodenal ulcers. What laboratory test should be ordered in the evaluation of the presumptive diagnosis?

64. A 76-year-old resident of a long-term care facility develops dysphagia and odynophagia. The medication list includes potassium chloride, vitamin C, and alendronate. An esophagogastroduodenoscopy reveals 2–3 discrete ulcers in the esophagus. In addition to taking medication with 4 oz water, what additional patient education is most appropriate to communicate regarding intake of these medications?

65. What over-the-counter medication, commonly taken by patients for noninflammatory diarrhea, may cause harmless black stools?

66. A 19-year-old college student presents to the university clinic with an acute onset of nausea, vomiting, and watery, non-bloody diarrhea. She attended an outdoor summer picnic 4 hours ago and consumed egg and potato salad. What is the etiologic agent associated with her infectious diarrhea?

(See answers next page.)

59. Empiric antibiotic

The clinical vignette supports the diagnosis of spontaneous bacterial peritonitis. Antibiotic therapy such as a third-generation cephalosporin, a combination beta-lactam/beta-lactamase agent, or a fluoroquinolone would be appropriate.

Blueprint Task: *Pharmaceutical Therapeutics*
Cognitive Level: *Analyze*

60. Squamous cell carcinoma

Squamous cell carcinoma is more common in individuals with a chronic history of tobacco and alcohol use, whereas a key characteristic of adenocarcinoma is the association with Barrett esophagus.

Blueprint Task: *Applying Basic Scientific Concepts*
Cognitive Level: *Apply*

61. Perforated gastric ulcer

The clinical vignette supports the diagnosis of a perforated gastric ulcer. Tobacco use interferes with ulcer healing and diminishes response to therapy.

Blueprint Task: *Formulating Most Likely Diagnosis*
Cognitive Level: *Apply*

62. Dysphagia

Dysphagia may occur with consumption of both solids and liquids. Gastroesophageal reflux disease may co-exist.

Blueprint Task: *History Taking and Performing Physical Examination*
Cognitive Level: *Apply*

63. Fasting gastrin level

The clinical vignette supports the diagnosis of Zollinger-Ellison Syndrome (ZES). ZES causes hypersecretion of gastrin which stimulates the release of hydrochloric acid by the parietal cells.

Blueprint Task: *Using Diagnostic and Laboratory Studies*
Cognitive Level: *Analyze*

64. Remain upright 30 minutes after ingestion

The clinical vignette supports the diagnosis of pill-induced esophagitis.

Blueprint Task: *Health Maintenance, Patient Education, and Preventive Measures*
Cognitive Level: *Analyze*

65. Bismuth subsalicylate

Blueprint Task: *Pharmaceutical Therapeutics*
Cognitive Level: *Recall*

66. *Staphylococcus aureus (S. aureus)*

The symptoms, incubation period, and food sources suggest infectious diarrhea caused by *S. aureus*.

Blueprint Task: *Formulating Most Likely Diagnosis*
Cognitive Level: *Apply*

67. A 23-year-old woman presents to the clinic with a 9-month history of intermittent lower abdominal pain, diarrhea, bloating, and flatulence. She denies fever, unintentional weight loss, or hematochezia. She has an unremarkable physical exam, and laboratory workup is negative. What is the most likely diagnosis?

68. A 63-year-old woman presents to the clinic with dysphagia to solids and liquids and regurgitation of food. A barium esophagram reveals a dilated esophagus with tapering at the gastroesophageal junction. What diagnostic study confirms the presumptive diagnosis?

69. What condition is defined by the replacement of normal squamous mucosa to metaplastic columnar epithelium in the distal esophagus?

70. A 57-year-old man with cirrhosis develops mild confusion and drowsiness. He has an elevated ammonia level. What two medications are known to improve this condition?

71. A 72-year-old man with atherosclerotic disease presents to the emergency department with an acute onset of severe abdominal pain. The pain is diffuse and worse after meals. He is without significant tenderness on exam. CT angiography reveals stenosis of the celiac and superior mesenteric arteries. What is the most likely diagnosis?

72. A 43-year-old woman presents to the clinic for evaluation of abnormal liver tests, specifically mildly elevated aminotransferases. She has a history of type 2 diabetes and hypertriglyceridemia with a BMI of 33 kg/m². She denies a history of alcohol use. Physical exam reveals right upper quadrant discomfort and hepatomegaly. What imaging study is most appropriate to support the presumptive diagnosis?

73. A 42-year-old woman with a BMI of 32 kg/m² presents to the emergency department with persistent right upper quadrant (RUQ) pain radiating to the right shoulder associated with nausea, vomiting, and fever. What specialized exam finding is associated with the presumptive diagnosis?

74. A patient is found to have the following lab findings: +HBsAg, +IgM Anti-HBc, –Anti-HBs. What is the presumptive diagnosis?

(See answers next page.)

67. Irritable bowel syndrome (IBS)

IBS is functional and multifactorial. The Rome IV criteria are used to establish the diagnosis.

Blueprint Task: *History Taking and Performing Physical Examination*

Cognitive Level: *Apply*

68. Esophageal manometry

The clinical vignette supports the diagnosis of achalasia. The findings on the barium esophagram represent a "bird's beak." Esophageal manometry confirms aperistalsis and impaired relaxation of the lower esophageal sphincter.

Blueprint Task: *Using Diagnostic and Laboratory Studies*

Cognitive Level: *Analyze*

69. Barrett esophagus

Blueprint Task: *Applying Basic Scientifi Concepts*

Cognitive Level: *Recall*

70. Lactulose and rifaximin

The clinical vignette supports a diagnosis of hepatic encephalopathy, a complication of cirrhosis. Both medications alter intestinal flora to reduce ammonia.

Blueprint Task: *Pharmaceutical Therapeutics*

Cognitive Level: *Analyze*

71. Acute mesenteric ischemia

The clinical vignette of acute severe postprandial abdominal pain that is out of proportion to the physical exam, coupled with the angiographic findings, support the diagnosis of acute mesenteric ischemia.

Blueprint Task: *Formulating Most Likely Diagnosis*

Cognitive Level: *Apply*

72. Ultrasound of liver

The clinical vignette supports the diagnosis of nonalcoholic fatty liver disease (NAFLD). Recommendations for a healthful diet, weight loss, and exercise management are appropriate.

Blueprint Task: *Using Diagnostic and Laboratory Studies*

Cognitive Level: *Analyze*

73. Murphy's sign

The clinical vignette supports the diagnosis of acute cholecystitis. Halting of inspiration due to pain from palpating the RUQ represents a positive Murphy's sign.

Blueprint Task: *History Taking and Performing Physical Examination*

Cognitive Level: *Analyze*

74. Acute hepatitis B infection

+HBsAg and +IgM Anti-HBc suggest active acute hepatitis B infection.

Blueprint Task: *Using Diagnostic and Laboratory Studies*

Cognitive Level: *Apply*

75. A 74-year-old man who takes daily opioids for severe osteoarthritis presents with generalized abdominal pain, nausea, and occasional liquid stool. The last bowel movement that he recalls was 1 week ago. His abdomen is mildly distended with mild diffuse discomfort on exam. Rectal exam reveals firm feces in the rectal vault. What is the most appropriate treatment for the presumptive diagnosis?

76. A 48-year-old woman with a history of injection drug use and high-risk sexual behaviors presents to the clinic with skin changes. On physical exam, she has small dilated blood vessels on her cheeks and nose, reddening of her palms, and dilated abdominal wall veins. The dermatologic manifestations are associated with what underlying condition?

77. A 6-year-old girl presents with abdominal pain that began in the epigastric area and now is localized to the right lower quadrant. She is febrile with right lower quadrant tenderness. A complete blood count shows a leukocytosis. What is the most appropriate initial imaging modality based on the presumptive diagnosis?

78. A 32-year-old man presents to the clinic with intermittent episodes of right lower quadrant abdominal pain, diarrhea, occasional aphthous ulcers, arthralgias, and a 10-pound unintentional weight loss over the last 6 months. Laboratory workup reveals iron and B12 deficiency anemia. He was recently treated for a perianal abscess. What is the presumptive diagnosis?

79. A 45-year-old man with type 2 diabetes and a recent HbA1c of 10.2% presents with odynophagia and dysphagia. An esophagogastroduodenoscopy (EGD) reveals white plaques lining the mucosa of the esophagus. What class of medication is most appropriate to treat the presumptive diagnosis?

80. A 34-year-old man presents to the clinic with a 3-month history of intermittent episodes of bloody diarrhea, abdominal cramping, and tenesmus. Sigmoidoscopy reveals friability and erosions extending from the rectum proximally to the sigmoid colon in a continuous circumferential pattern. What is the most likely diagnosis?

81. A 54-year-old man with a history of peptic ulcer disease (PUD) presents with epigastric abdominal pain, nausea, early satiety, vomiting, and gastric distention. What physical exam finding represents a complication of this condition?

(See answers next page.)

75. Enema
The clinical vignette supports the diagnosis of fecal impaction. Enemas containing mineral oil or saline can be utilized, and if bowel movement does not occur, digital disruption can be performed.
Blueprint Task: *Clinical Intervention*
Cognitive Level: *Analyze*

76. Cirrhosis
Dermatologic manifestations such as jaundice, spider telangiectasias, palmar erythema, and caput medusae may be seen with cirrhosis. Cirrhosis results from conditions such as hepatitis B and C virus.
Blueprint Task: *History Taking and Performing Physical Examination*
Cognitive Level: *Analyze*

77. Ultrasound
The clinical vignette supports the diagnosis of acute appendicitis, and ultrasound is the imaging tool of choice in children and nonobese, young adults.
Blueprint Task: *Using Diagnostic and Laboratory Studies*
Cognitive Level: *Analyze*

78. Crohn disease
The clinical vignette, including intestinal and extraintestinal symptoms with perianal disease, supports the diagnosis of Crohn disease. Crohn disease may present with skip lesions anywhere from the mouth to anus and may cause penetrating, fistulizing disease
Blueprint Task: *Formulating Most Likely Diagnosis*
Cognitive Level: *Apply*

79. Antifungal
The clinical vignette supports the diagnosis of candida esophagitis which is more common in an immunocompromised patient. Fluconazole is the most commonly prescribed oral antifungal medication.
Blueprint Task: *Pharmaceutical Therapeutics*
Cognitive Level: *Analyze*

80. Ulcerative colitis
The clinical vignette supports the diagnosis of ulcerative colitis. Ulcerative colitis exclusively involves the colon.
Blueprint Task: *Formulating Most Likely Diagnosis*
Cognitive Level: *Apply*

81. Succussion splash
The clinical vignette supports a gastric outlet obstruction, which can present with a succussion splash. Other complications of PUD include hemorrhage and perforation, which can manifest as hematemesis or melena and with peritoneal signs, respectively.
Blueprint Task: *History Taking and Performing Physical Examination*
Cognitive Level: *Analyze*

82. A 50-year-old man presents with an 8-week history of change in bowel habits. Previously, he had one formed stool daily and currently reports episodes of loose stools and colicky lower abdominal discomfort. He reports daily heavy alcohol use for the last 10 years with a diet high in red and processed meats and low in fruits and vegetables. The patient notes blood-streaked stools in the past month, and the stool guaiac is positive. The physical exam is otherwise normal. What is the most likely diagnosis?

83. What condition may be visualized by inspecting the abdomen while the patient actively lifts head and shoulders off the examination table?

84. A 22-year-old woman is referred to the gastroenterologist for iron deficiency anemia. An esophagogastroduodenoscopy (EGD) with duodenal biopsies reveals intraepithelial lymphocytosis and villous atrophy. What is the most likely diagnosis?

85. A 47-year-old woman with a history of multiple abdominal surgeries presents to the emergency department with nausea, vomiting, and obstipation. On physical exam, she has a distended, tympanic abdomen. Supine and upright abdominal x-rays reveal dilated loops of bowel with differential air-fluid levels. What nonpharmacological intervention is recommended to provide relief of symptoms?

86. A patient with a history of retching and hematemesis has a laceration at the gastroesophageal junction on esophagogastroduodenoscopy. What additional historical factor is common in a patient with this presumptive diagnosis?

(*See answers next page.*)

82. Colon cancer
The clinical vignette supports the diagnosis of left-sided colon cancer based on the patient's age, history of alcohol use, and poor diet, along with symptoms of hematochezia and bowel changes.
Blueprint Task: Formulating Most Likely Diagnosis
Cognitive Level: Analyze

83. Abdominal wall (ventral) hernia
Blueprint Task: History Taking and Performing Physical Examination
Cognitive Level: Recall

84. Celiac disease
The clinical vignette and duodenal findings support a diagnosis of Celiac disease, which can cause malabsorption.
Blueprint Task: Formulating Most Likely Diagnosis
Cognitive Level: Apply

85. Nasogastric (NG) tube to suction
The clinical vignette supports the diagnosis of small bowel obstruction (SBO). Adhesions are the most common cause of SBO. Additional management may include NPO status, IV fluid therapy, electrolyte replacement, anti-emetic therapy, and surgery consult.
Blueprint Task: Clinical Intervention
Cognitive Level: Analyze

86. Heavy alcohol use
The clinical vignette supports the diagnosis of Mallory–Weiss tear.
Blueprint Task: History Taking and Performing Physical Examination
Cognitive Level: Analyze

Genitourinary System (Male and Female)

1. In a patient with testicular pain, relief of pain upon elevation of the scrotum describes what sign?

2. A 41-year-old woman with a BMI of 32 kg/m² presents to the clinic with involuntary leakage of urine during exercising, laughing, and sneezing. In addition to encouraging weight loss and dietary changes, what exercise is initially recommended to improve symptoms associated with the presumptive diagnosis?

3. A 65-year-old man presents to the clinic with nocturia, urinary hesitancy, dribbling, weak stream, and incomplete bladder emptying. Physical exam reveals a smooth, enlarged prostate without tenderness or nodules. What class of medication would be most appropriate to decrease the size of the prostate?

4. A 19-year-old woman presents to the clinic with a 2-day history of dysuria, frequency, and urgency. She has mild suprapubic tenderness but no costovertebral angle tenderness, fever, or vaginal discharge. She is not sexually active. What is the most likely pathogen causing the presumptive diagnosis?

5. What three serum tumor markers may be associated with testicular cancer?

6. A 72-year-old woman with a history of multiple vaginal births presents to the clinic with urinary urgency and incontinence. She is initiated on an antimuscarinic medication. What ocular side effect may be associated with this pharmaceutical class?

7. What newborn physical exam finding presents as a ventral displacement of the urethral meatus and should delay elective circumcision?

8. A 28-year-old woman presents to the clinic with recurrent postcoital urinary tract infections. Besides treatment with an appropriate antibiotic following intercourse, what recommended routine self-care practice can also help to decrease recurrences?

1. Prehn sign

Blueprint Task: History Taking and Performing Physical Examination
Cognitive Level: Recall

2. Kegel

The clinical vignette supports the diagnosis of stress urinary incontinence (SUI). Kegel exercises strengthen pelvic floor muscles.

Blueprint Task: Health Maintenance, Patient Education, and Preventive Measures
Cognitive Level: Analyze

3. 5-Alpha-reductase inhibitors

The clinical vignette supports the diagnosis of benign prostatic hyperplasia. 5-alpha reductase inhibitors reduce the prostate size via antiandrogen effects.

Blueprint Task: Pharmaceutical Therapeutics
Cognitive Level: Apply

4. *Escherichia coli* (*E. coli*)

The clinical vignette supports the diagnosis of cystitis

Blueprint Task: Applying Basic Scientific Concepts
Cognitive Level: Analyze

5. Alpha-fetoprotein (AFP), beta subunit of the human chorionic gonadotropin (beta-hCG), and lactate dehydrogenase (LDH)

Blueprint Task: Using Diagnostic and Laboratory Studies
Cognitive Level: Recall

6. Blurred vision

Antimuscarinics can contribute to additional anticholinergic side effects such as dry mouth, constipation, and other issues. These side effects may limit drug tolerability and escalation of therapy.

Blueprint Task: Pharmaceutical Therapeutics
Cognitive Level: Apply

7. Hypospadias

Hypospadias is a fairly common genitourinary finding and complicates the use of standard devices for circumcision. Delay in circumcision is also recommended to preserve the foreskin tissue for use during the surgical repair of this defect.

Blueprint Task: History Taking and Performing Physical Examination
Cognitive Level: Apply

8. Postcoital urinary voiding

Blueprint Task: Health Maintenance, Patient Education, and Preventive Measures
Cognitive Level: Recall

9. A 45-year-old man presents to the clinic with concerns of "heaviness" and asymmetry in the right groin for the past several months. His symptoms are more pronounced when he coughs and strains. On physical exam, an abnormal bulge is recognized upon Valsalva maneuver and reduces easily. What is the most likely diagnosis?

10. A 12-year-old boy presents to the emergency department with his parents reporting an abrupt onset of severe, persistent left-sided scrotal pain that awoke him 1 hour ago. He is nauseated and has vomited twice. The scrotum is swollen, erythematous, and the cremasteric reflex is absent. What emergent imaging study will provide the definitive diagnosis?

11. What is the most commonly used class of medication prescribed for erectile dysfunction that is contraindicated in patients taking nitroglycerine?

12. What is the most common type of bladder cancer?

13. What endocrine disorder can contribute to the development of renal stones?

14. A 25-year-old woman presents with a 3-day history of worsening dysuria, frequency, and urgency. In the last 24 hours, she has developed a fever of 38.3°C (101°F) and flank pain. She has no history of nephrolithiasis. What type of urinary cast on urine microscopy is associated with the presumptive diagnosis?

15. A 55-year-old man with a history of urethral stricture presents to the clinic with 2 days of urinary urgency, frequency, dysuria, and perineal pain. He denies hematuria, flank and testicular pain, and urethral discharge. On physical exam, the patient is febrile with an enlarged, edematous, and tender prostate. What is the most likely diagnosis?

16. A 69-year-old man with a long-standing history of tobacco use and employment in the textile industry has had persistent microscopic hematuria for years. He has previously declined a workup for hematuria. He denies dysuria and is not taking any medication. What is the recommended procedure for confirmation of the most likely diagnosis?

(See answers next page.)

9. Inguinal hernia

Indirect inguinal is the most common type of hernia and travels through the inguinal canal. Direct inguinal hernias protrude through Hesselbach's triangle. Incarcerated or strangulated hernias require urgent repair.

Blueprint Task: *Formulating Most Likely Diagnosis*
Cognitive Level: *Apply*

10. Color doppler ultrasound of the scrotum

The clinical vignette supports the diagnosis of testicular torsion. Imaging studies should not delay emergent urologic referral.

Blueprint Task: *Clinical Intervention*
Cognitive Level: *Analyze*

11. Phosphodiesterase-5 (PDE5) inhibitors

The risk of nitroglycerine use with PDE5 inhibitors is due to vasodilation and may lead to hypotension and syncope.

Blueprint Task: *Pharmaceutical Therapeutics*
Cognitive Level: *Apply*

12. Urothelial cell carcinoma (transitional cell carcinoma)

Blueprint Task: *Applying Basic Scientific Concepts*
Cognitive Level: *Recall*

13. Primary hyperparathyroidism

Primary hyperparathyroidism can cause hypercalcemia. Most renal stones are of calcium composition.

Blueprint Task: *History Taking and Performing Physical Examination*
Cognitive Level: *Apply*

14. White blood cell (WBC) cast

The clinical vignette supports the diagnosis of pyelonephritis

Blueprint Task: *Using Diagnostic and Laboratory Studies*
Cognitive Level: *Analyze*

15. Acute prostatitis

Acute prostatitis may be caused by factors such as recent urogenital instrumentation and urinary tract abnormalities (e.g., urethral stricture).

Blueprint Task: *Formulating Most Likely Diagnosis*
Cognitive Level: *Apply*

16. Cystoscopy

The clinical vignette supports the diagnosis of bladder cancer. Key historical features include persistent hematuria, tobacco history, and exposure to occupational hazards. Urine cytology may also be helpful in the evaluation.

Blueprint Task: *Clinical Intervention*
Cognitive Level: *Analyze*

17. In a newborn with epispadias, what is the abnormal position of the urethral meatus?

18. A 45-year-old woman presents to the clinic with a 6-month history of intermittent episodes of urinary urgency, frequency, dysuria, and suprapubic tenderness. Symptoms worsen with bladder filling and improve with voiding. With each episode, a urine microscopy and culture are unremarkable. A cystoscopy reveals petechial hemorrhages. What medication helps to reconstitute the glycosaminoglycan layer of the urothelium in the treatment of the presumptive diagnosis?

19. What viral infection may precede the development of parotitis and orchitis?

20. A patient with cystitis is prescribed an antibiotic as well as phenazopyridine for symptomatic relief. If the patient is a contact lens wearer, what education is important to share related to a common side effect of phenazopyridine?

21. A 35-year-old man with a recent spinal cord injury is evaluated for recurrent urinary tract infections. He relays that he cannot sense when his bladder is full and frequently has urinary incontinence. What diagnostic intervention may support the cause for his recurrent urinary tract infections?

22. A 64-year-old man presents to the clinic with sexual dysfunction. He reports painful erections and abnormal curvature of the penis. The physical exam reveals thickening of the dorsum of the penis. What is the most likely diagnosis?

23. What physical exam test is performed by stroking the inner thigh and assessing for elevation of the ipsilateral testes?

24. A 9-year-old girl presents to the clinic for bloody spotting in her underwear and mild pain with wiping following urination. The mother describes a history of chronic constipation and difficulty with urination. Sitz baths have provided minimal relief. Physical exam of the urethra reveals a protruding doughnut-shaped mass. Urinalysis is unremarkable. What pharmacologic therapy is recommended for the presumptive diagnosis?

25. What is the name of the condition that results in the inability to retract the foreskin of the penis?

(See answers next page.)

17. Dorsal
Blueprint Task: *Applying Basic Scientific Concepts*
Cognitive Level: *Recall*

18. Pentosan polysulfate
The clinical vignette supports the diagnosis of interstitial cystitis.
Blueprint Task: *Pharmaceutical Therapeutics*
Cognitive Level: *Analyze*

19. Mumps
Blueprint Task: *History Taking and Performing Physical Examination*
Cognitive Level: *Recall*

20. Possible staining of contact lens
Phenazopyridine causes an orange discoloration of bodily fluids, including tears and may stain contact lens.
Blueprint Task: *Health Maintenance, Patient Education, and Preventive Measures*
Cognitive Level: *Apply*

21. Measurement of post-void residual volume
The clinical vignette supports the diagnosis of urinary retention secondary to neurogenic bladder, which can be found in patients with spinal cord injury. A bladder ultrasound with catheterization allows for measurement of post-void residual volume.
Blueprint Task: *Using Diagnostic and Laboratory Studies*
Cognitive Level: *Analyze*

22. Peyronie's disease
The pathophysiologic cause of Peyronie's disease is multifactorial and commonly attributed to tunica albuginea fibrosis. Patients may report difficulty with intercourse due to deformity.
Blueprint Task: *Formulating Most Likely Diagnosis*
Cognitive Level: *Apply*

23. Cremasteric reflex
Blueprint Task: *History Taking and Performing Physical Examination*
Cognitive Level: *Recall*

24. Topical estrogen cream
The clinical vignette supports the diagnosis of urethral prolapse. Sitz baths may be therapeutic in addition to topical estrogen cream. Rarely surgical intervention may be required.
Blueprint Task: *Clinical Intervention*
Cognitive Level: *Analyze*

25. Phimosis
Blueprint Task: *Applying Basic Scientific Concepts*
Cognitive Level: *Recall*

26. A patient is found to have an elevated prostate-specific antigen (PSA) and a firm mass on the prostate. What diagnostic intervention is utilized to confirm the presumptive diagnosis?

27. A 50-year-old man presents to the emergency department with persistent penile erection for the past 4 hours. He reports no recent history of sexual activity or penile stimulation. What is the most likely diagnosis?

28. A 22-year-old uncircumcised man with type 1 diabetes presents to the clinic with erythema and tenderness of the glans penis, along with a white curd-like substance under the foreskin. What is the most appropriate treatment for the presumptive diagnosis?

29. What is the name of an abnormal curvature of the penis that may be associated with hypospadias?

30. A 7-month-old infant presents with his mother as a new patient and is determined to have an undescended left testes since birth. There are no other abnormal findings on the physical exam. What is the recommended management for the presumptive diagnosis?

31. What viral infection can contribute to the development of penile cancer?

32. What laboratory test is utilized for prostate cancer screening but may also be elevated in benign prostatic hyperplasia and prostatitis?

33. A 16-year-old adolescent presents for his sports physical. On inguinal hernia exam, he is found to have left-sided scrotal fullness with engorged vessels. What is the presumptive diagnosis?

34. A 56-year-old woman with a BMI of 32 kg/m^2, multiple vaginal births, and chronic constipation presents with involuntary leakage of urine, dyspareunia, and the sensation of a bulge in the vagina. Physical exam reveals a cystocele. What is the most likely diagnosis?

(*See answers next page.*)

26. Transrectal ultrasound-guided biopsy

The clinical vignette supports the diagnosis of prostate cancer.

Blueprint Task: Using Diagnostic and Laboratory Studies
Cognitive Level: Apply

27. Priapism

Priapism is a urologic emergency due to risk of tissue ischemia.

Blueprint Task: Formulating Most Likely Diagnosis
Cognitive Level: Apply

28. Topical antifungal

The clinical vignette supports the diagnosis of balanitis secondary to candida infection. Infection with bacteria may necessitate the use of antibiotics.

Blueprint Task: Pharmaceutical Therapeutics
Cognitive Level: Analyze

29. Chordee

Blueprint Task: History Taking and Performing Physical Examination
Cognitive Level: Recall

30. Referral to pediatric urology for possible orchiopexy

The clinical vignette supports the diagnosis of cryptorchidism. Spontaneous descent is rare after 4–6 months of age. Potential complications of cryptorchidism include decreased fertility and testicular cancer.

Blueprint Task: Clinical Intervention
Cognitive Level: Apply

31. Human papillomavirus (HPV)

Blueprint Task: Applying Basic Scientific Concepts
Cognitive Level: Recall

32. Prostate-specific antigen (PSA)

Blueprint Task: Using Diagnostic and Laboratory Studies
Cognitive Level: Recall

33. Varicocele

The clinical vignette supports the diagnosis of a varicocele often described as a "bag of worms".

Blueprint Task: Formulating Most Likely Diagnosis
Cognitive Level: Apply

34. Pelvic organ prolapse

Pelvic organ prolapse may be associated with risk factors such as elevated BMI, multiple births, advancing age, and chronic constipation.

Blueprint Task: History Taking and Performing Physical Examination
Cognitive Level: Apply

35. A patient presents to the office with weak urinary stream and incomplete emptying. He is found to have fibrosis of the urethra and has undergone endoscopic dilation without improvement. What treatment is now recommended for the presumptive diagnosis?

36. What class of medication may alleviate lower urinary tract symptoms associated with benign prostatic hyperplasia but can lead to hypotension?

37. A 9-month-old girl is diagnosed with recurrent urinary tract infections (UTIs). The cause of the UTIs is believed to be due to the abnormal flow of urine from the bladder up toward the kidney during voiding. What imaging study is recommended to confirm the most likely diagnosis?

38. What is the most common sexual desire disorder affecting both men and women?

39. A 55-year-old woman with severe diverticular disease presents to the clinic with irritative voiding symptoms, pneumaturia, and fecaluria. Urinalysis reveals pyuria and bacteriuria. What potential complication of diverticular disease is this patient most likely experiencing?

40. A 42-year-old woman was thrown off a horse and sustained a direct blow to the low abdomen and pelvis. She is experiencing significant suprapubic pain and hematuria. Physical exam reveals severe lower abdominal tenderness. Radiograph of the pelvis reveals pelvic fracture. What additional diagnosis, associated with the pelvic fracture, is most likely in this patient?

41. An 8-year-old girl presents with her mother for recurrent episodes of urinary frequency and dysuria. Urinalysis is normal. The patient's mother reports that her daughter likes to take bubble baths daily. What is the presumptive diagnosis?

42. A 55-year-old man with an allergy to sulfa requires treatment for acute bacterial prostatitis. What medication class is most appropriate?

43. A newborn presents to the clinic with painless swelling and enlargement of the scrotum. On physical exam, the left scrotum transilluminates. What is the most likely diagnosis?

(See answers next page.)

35. Urethroplasty

The clinical vignette supports the diagnosis of urethral stricture. After failed endoscopic therapy, surgical therapy is typically recommended.

Blueprint Task: *Clinical Intervention*
Cognitive Level: *Analyze*

36. Alpha-adrenergic receptor antagonists

Blueprint Task: *Pharmaceutical Therapeutics*
Cognitive Level: *Recall*

37. Voiding cystourethrogram (VCUG)

The clinical vignette supports the diagnosis of vesicoureteral reflux.

Blueprint Task: *Using Diagnostic and Laboratory Studies*
Cognitive Level: *Analyze*

38. Hypoactive sexual desire disorder (HSSD)

Blueprint Task: *Formulating Most Likely Diagnosis*
Cognitive Level: *Recall*

39. Colovesical fistula

Colovesical fistula can occur in patients with complicated diverticular disease.

Blueprint Task: *History Taking and Performing Physical Examination*
Cognitive Level: *Apply*

40. Bladder rupture

The review of systems in patients with pelvic trauma should include bladder symptom questioning. Full bladder at time of pelvic trauma increases risk of bladder rupture.

Blueprint Task: *Formulating Most Likely Diagnosis*
Cognitive Level: *Apply*

41. Chemical urethritis

Blueprint Task: *Health Maintenance, Patient Education, and Preventive Measures*
Cognitive Level: *Recall*

42. Fluoroquinolones

Although fluoroquinolones or trimethoprim/sulfamethoxazole (TMP-SMX) can be used in the treatment of acute bacterial prostatitis, TMP-SMX is avoided in this patient due to his sulfa allergy.

Blueprint Task: *Pharmaceutical Therapeutics*
Cognitive Level: *Apply*

43. Hydrocele

Blueprint Task: *History Taking and Performing Physical Examination*
Cognitive Level: *Recall*

44. A 21-year-old woman presents to the clinic with a 2-day history of urinary urgency, frequency, dysuria, and suprapubic tenderness. She is not sexually active and is without vaginal symptoms or flank and pelvic pain. Urine dipstick is positive for leukocyte esterase and nitrites. What is the most likely diagnosis?

45. What is an intravaginal device used for genital prolapse that may also be beneficial in patients with stress urinary incontinence?

46. What emergent condition may be avoided by advising new parents against aggressive foreskin retraction and to return the foreskin to a natural position after bathing an uncircumcised newborn?

47. What urologic procedure used in symptomatic nephrolithiasis, unresponsive to conservative management, involves directed transmission of high energy to encourage fragmentation and spontaneous passage of stone?

48. A 55-year-old man presents to the clinic with irritative voiding symptoms and scrotal pain. He is in a monogamous relationship. Physical exam reveals erythema, edema, and tenderness of the left scrotal sac, which improves with elevation. There are no penile lesions or urethral discharge. What is the most likely diagnosis?

(See answers next page.)

44. Acute simple cystitis

The clinical vignette describes acute simple cystitis given the presence of irritative voiding symptoms and positive dipstick results to support infection.

Blueprint Task: Formulating Most Likely Diagnosis
Cognitive Level: Apply

45. Pessary

Blueprint Task: Clinical Intervention
Cognitive Level: Recall

46. Paraphimosis

Paraphimosis is a urologic emergency as, without treatment, it may lead to ischemia and tissue destruction.

Blueprint Task: Health Maintenance, Patient Education, and Preventive Measures
Cognitive Level: Apply

47. Extracorporeal shock wave lithotripsy

Blueprint Task: Clinical Intervention
Cognitive Level: Recall

48. Epididymitis

Epididymitis presents with a unilateral tender and swollen epididymitis with or without urethritis. Prehn sign helps distinguish epididymitis from testicular torsion.

Blueprint Task: Formulating Most Likely Diagnosis
Cognitive Level: Apply

Hematologic System

1. On physical exam, a patient is found to have hemarthrosis and ecchymosis, which he reports has been a recurrent problem since childhood. Laboratory evaluation reveals prolonged aPTT and normal PT. What factor deficiency is the cause of the presumptive diagnosis?

2. What is the expected increase in hemoglobin and hematocrit in an adult patient receiving one unit of packed red blood cells?

3. A 62-year-old man presents to the clinic with abnormal episodes of epistaxis and gingival bleeding over the last week. He also describes bone pain that awakens him at night. Physical exam reveals pallor with purpura and petechiae. Cytology confirms the presence of Auer rods. What is the most likely diagnosis?

4. A 23-year-old man with sickle cell disease recently started a job as a lifeguard. What risk factor may precipitate a pain crisis given his new occupation?

5. What is the approximate life span of a red blood cell?

6. A 65-year-old man has a malignancy of plasma cells characterized by bone pain, fatigue, and radiographic lytic lesions. What would be the expected finding on serum protein electrophoresis?

7. What clinical intervention should be considered in a patient presenting with autoimmune hemolytic anemia refractory to pharmacologic therapy?

8. What medication is commonly given prophylactically to high-risk hospitalized patients to lower the potential of developing a deep vein thrombosis?

9. A 20-year-old woman with no chronic medical problems is found to have iron-deficiency anemia. She reports mild fatigue. She has a consistent nutritious dietary intake and denies melena or hematochezia. The physical exam is normal. What historical feature is important to elicit to determine the most likely cause of her iron-deficiency anemia?

1. Factor VIII deficiency
The clinical vignette supports the diagnosis of hemophilia A, a genetic coagulation disorder that results in bleeding due to Factor VIII deficiency.
Blueprint Task: History Taking and Performing Physical Examination
Cognitive Level: Analyze

2. Hemoglobin by 1 g/dL and hematocrit by 3%
Blueprint Task: Clinical Intervention
Cognitive Level: Recall

3. Acute myeloid leukemia (AML)
The laboratory finding of Auer rods is pathognomonic for AML.
Blueprint Task: Formulating Most Likely Diagnosis
Cognitive Level: Apply

4. Dehydration
Additional risk factors for the development of vaso-occlusive crises include infection, sudden temperature change, and hypoxia.
Blueprint Task: Health Maintenance, Patient Education, and Preventive Measures
Cognitive Level: Apply

5. 120 days
Blueprint Task: Applying Basic Scientific Concepts
Cognitive Level: Recall

6. Paraprotein with monoclonal spike
The clinical vignette supports the diagnosis of plasma cell myeloma (formerly termed multiple myeloma).
Blueprint Task: Using Diagnostic and Laboratory Studies
Cognitive Level: Analyze

7. Splenectomy
Common pharmacologic therapies include glucocorticoids or rituximab.
Blueprint Task: Clinical Intervention
Cognitive Level: Apply

8. Heparin
Blueprint Task: Pharmaceutical Therapeutics
Cognitive Level: Recall

9. Heavy menses
Chronic blood loss is a common cause of iron-deficiency anemia. It is essential to obtain a thorough menstrual history, including duration, frequency, and flow of menstrual cycle
Blueprint Task: History Taking and Performing Physical Examination
Cognitive Level: Apply

10. What common over-the-counter medication affects the function of platelets by impairing platelet aggregation?

11. A healthy 5-year-old girl presents to the office with diffuse petechial rash, areas of ecchymosis, and an episode of epistaxis. She had a recent mild viral upper respiratory infection but is now feeling better. The complete blood count is normal except for a platelet count of 30,000 mm³. What is the presumptive diagnosis?

12. What would be the expected aPTT and PT findings in a patient with hemophilia B?

13. In a patient with pernicious anemia due to lack of intrinsic factor, what clinical intervention is recommended to demonstrate gastric atrophy?

14. What term describes immature red blood cells?

15. A 56-year-old man presents to the clinic with fatigue. On physical exam, his nails appear fragile and spoon-shaped. This abnormal nail finding is most likely associated with what hematologic condition?

16. What is the most common pediatric cancer and is characterized by pancytopenia with circulating blasts?

17. A 24-year-old man presents to the clinic with right upper quadrant pain and is found to have non-obstructive gallstones and splenomegaly. Laboratory studies reveal a mild, normocytic anemia with an increased mean corpuscular hemoglobin concentration, normal red blood cell count, slightly elevated bilirubin, and normal liver enzymes. Peripheral blood smear shows numerous spherocytes. What is the presumptive diagnosis?

18. What is the definition of anisocytosis?

(See answers next page.)

10. Aspirin

Blueprint Task: Health Maintenance, Patient Education, and Preventive Measures
Cognitive Level: Recall

11. Immune thrombocytopenia (ITP)

ITP (formerly termed idiopathic thrombocytopenic purpura) is an autoimmune-mediated clearance of platelets. It is the most common bleeding disorder of childhood and often is associated with an antecedent viral infection.

Blueprint Task: Formulating Most Likely Diagnosis
Cognitive Level: Analyze

12. Prolonged aPTT; normal PT

Hemophilia B, also called Christmas disease, is due to Factor IX deficiency.

Blueprint Task: Using Diagnostic and Laboratory Studies
Cognitive Level: Apply

13. Endoscopy with gastric biopsy

Endoscopy with biopsy will show gastric atrophy of all the layers of the body and fundus.

Blueprint Task: Clinical Intervention
Cognitive Level: Apply

14. Reticulocytes

Blueprint Task: Applying Basic Scientific Concepts
Cognitive Level: Recall

15. Iron-deficiency anemia

The described nail findings represent koilonychia.

Blueprint Task: History Taking and Performing Physical Examination
Cognitive Level: Apply

16. Acute lymphoblastic leukemia (ALL)

Blueprint Task: Using Diagnostic and Laboratory Studies
Cognitive Level: Recall

17. Hereditary spherocytosis

Hereditary spherocytosis can present in infancy as a significant anemia or as an adult with mild to moderate hemolytic anemia. Intermittent jaundice may also be present.

Blueprint Task: Formulating Most Likely Diagnosis
Cognitive Level: Apply

18. Variation of red blood cell size

Blueprint Task: Applying Basic Scientific Concepts
Cognitive Level: Recall

19. A 45-year-old man who works in the auto repair industry presents to the clinic with abdominal pain, constipation, vomiting, and generalized muscle pain for the past week. Labs reveal a microcytic anemia with basophilic stippling of erythrocytes. A bone marrow biopsy shows sideroblasts. What is the presumptive diagnosis?

20. What are the components of Virchow's triad?

21. What is the first-line pharmacologic therapy recommended for patients with von Willebrand disease (VWD) who are experiencing mild bleeding?

22. What vitamin taken with iron supplementation enhances absorption?

23. What autoimmune hematologic disease, either primary or associated with conditions such as systemic lupus erythematosus (SLE), is the most likely cause of recurrent clotting and pregnancy loss?

24. Which cell line on a complete blood count (CBC) would you expect to see elevated with a parasitic infection?

25. An asymptomatic 16-year-old girl with no known health problems and normal menses presents for a well-check visit. Labs reveal a mildly decreased hemoglobin and hematocrit, mildly decreased red blood cell count, low ferritin, low serum iron, and high total iron-binding capacity. The remainder of her lab work is normal. What is the recommended intervention for this patient?

26. What class of medication improves survival rate and is standard therapy for patients with chronic myeloid leukemia (CML)?

27. What nutrient deficiency is associated with pernicious anemia?

(See answers next page.)

19. Sideroblastic anemia

The sideroblastic anemia is most likely due to lead poisoning associated with the patient's high-risk occupation.

Blueprint Task: *Formulating Most Likely Diagnosis*
Cognitive Level: *Analyze*

20. Stasis, hypercoagulability, and vessel wall injury

Blueprint Task: *Applying Basic Scientific Concepts*
Cognitive Level: *Recall*

21. Desmopressin

Desmopressin is appropriate for mild bleeding; however, von Willebrand factor (VWF) concentrates are recommended for severe bleeding.

Blueprint Task: *Pharmaceutical Therapeutics*
Cognitive Level: *Apply*

22. Vitamin C (ascorbic acid)

Blueprint Task: *Health Maintenance, Patient Education, and Preventive Measures*
Cognitive Level: *Recall*

23. Antiphospholipid syndrome

Thrombosis is common in patients with antiphospholipid syndrome; as such, anticoagulation is a primary aspect of treatment.

Blueprint Task: *History Taking and Performing Physical Examination*
Cognitive Level: *Apply*

24. Eosinophils

Blueprint Task: *Using Diagnostic and Laboratory Studies*
Cognitive Level: *Recall*

25. Daily oral iron replacement

The clinical vignette supports the diagnosis of iron-deficiency anemia, which more commonly occurs in adolescence due to inadequate intake during rapid growth when not caused by dysfunctional uterine bleeding or menorrhagia.

Blueprint Task: *Clinical Intervention*
Cognitive Level: *Analyze*

26. Tyrosine kinase inhibitor (TKI)

Blueprint Task: *Pharmaceutical Therapeutics*
Cognitive Level: *Recall*

27. Vitamin B12

Blueprint Task: *Applying Basic Scientific Concepts*
Cognitive Level: *Recall*

28. What is the typical dermatologic finding associated with IgA vasculitis?

29. What is the major iron storage protein and is used in the diagnosis of iron-deficiency anemia?

30. A healthy 73-year-old man presents for medical clearance with routine blood work prior to a planned procedure for chronic back pain. The physical exam is consistent with his ongoing back condition but also reveals painless cervical lymphadenopathy. Labs reveal leukocytosis with a high percentage of small mature lymphocytes. What is your presumptive diagnosis?

31. A patient with hereditary thrombophilia has the highest risk of developing what potential complication?

32. A 26-year-old woman with meningitis and secondary sepsis shows indications of hypercoagulation to include signs of ischemia-related organ failure and thrombotic purpura. There is currently no sign of active bleeding, and the patient's platelet count is 40,000 mm^3. What clinical intervention would aid in reducing the risk of further thrombosis?

33. What pharmacologic therapy should be initiated emergently in a patient presenting with febrile neutropenia?

34. What would be the expected physical exam finding of the palpebral conjunctiva in a patient with severe anemia?

35. A patient with rheumatoid arthritis (RA) has neutropenia and splenomegaly. What syndrome do these signs represent?

36. Hospitalized patients with COVID-19 should receive what prophylactic intervention for associated thromboinflammation?

(*See answers next page.*)

28. Palpable purpura

Purpuric skin lesions are classically seen on the lower extremities and buttocks. IgA vasculitis was formerly termed Henoch-Schönlein purpura.

Blueprint Task: History Taking and Performing Physical Examination

Cognitive Level: Apply

29. Ferritin

Blueprint Task: Using Diagnostic and Laboratory Studies

Cognitive Level: Recall

30. Chronic lymphocytic leukemia (CLL)

Most patients with CLL are asymptomatic and are diagnosed incidentally during routine blood work.

Blueprint Task: Formulating Most Likely Diagnosis

Cognitive Level: Apply

31. Venous thromboembolism

Blueprint Task: Health Maintenance, Patient Education, and Preventive Measures

Cognitive Level: Recall

32. Low molecular weight heparin

The clinical vignette supports the diagnosis of disseminated intravascular coagulopathy. In patients at risk for thrombosis, with no active bleeding and platelet counts >30,000 mm3, low molecular weight heparin is recommended.

Blueprint Task: Clinical Intervention

Cognitive Level: Analyze

33. Empiric antibiotics

Febrile neutropenia is defined by a fever of >38°C (100.4°F) and an absolute neutrophil count (ANC) of 500 or less.

Blueprint Task: Pharmaceutical Therapeutics

Cognitive Level: Apply

34. Pallor

Blueprint Task: History Taking and Performing Physical Examination

Cognitive Level: Recall

35. Felty syndrome

RA associated with Felty syndrome is typically severe and erosive. Neutropenia increases the risk of infection.

Blueprint Task: Formulating Most Likely Diagnosis

Cognitive Level: Apply

36. Anticoagulation

Patients with more severe symptoms requiring hospitalization are at higher risk for venous thromboembolism, ischemic stroke, and myocardial infarction due to COVID-19-induced coagulopathy.

Blueprint Task: Clinical Intervention

Cognitive Level: Apply

37. A 22-year-old man presents to the clinic with fatigue, weight loss, night sweats, and fever. On physical exam, he has cervical lymphadenopathy and hepatomegaly. Hodgkin lymphoma is suspected. What characteristic multinucleated B cells found on lymph node biopsy confirm this diagnosis?

38. Sepsis is the leading cause of death in children with sickle cell anemia due to functional asplenia. What medication is typically given prophylactically to reduce the incidence of sepsis?

39. What is the term for a well-documented manifestation of iron deficiency involving the desire to consume non-nutritive substances such as clay, ice, and dirt?

40. A 14-year-old presents to the clinic with excessively heavy menstrual periods since menarche. She has experienced easy bruising and recurrent epistaxis with family history of similar symptoms. Laboratory evaluation reveals prolonged bleeding time and normal platelet count. What is the presumptive diagnosis?

41. A 65-year-old man presents to the clinic with progressive headaches, dizziness, tinnitus, fatigue, and bothersome pruritus after bathing. The patient has flushed skin and splenomegaly. Complete blood count reveals elevated hematocrit, white blood cells (WBC), and platelet counts. Red blood cells, WBC, and platelet morphology are normal. The presumptive diagnosis is confirmed with Janus Kinase 2 gene (JAK2) mutation screening. What is the treatment of choice for the presumptive diagnosis?

42. If medical treatment is necessary, what is the first-line class of pharmacologic therapy recommended for patients with immune thrombocytopenia (ITP)?

43. What is the most common hereditary thrombophilia in the United States?

44. A 7-year-old boy presents to the clinic with progressive purpuric rash to the buttocks and legs, intermittent sharp abdominal pain, and arthralgias in the ankles and knees over the last 2 days. He had a recent viral upper respiratory infection. Laboratory evaluation reveals a normal complete blood count, and urinalysis shows hematuria and proteinuria. What is the most likely diagnosis?

45. Thrombotic thrombocytopenic purpura (TTP) is associated with a classic pentad, although all five components are only seen in a small percentage of cases. The pentad includes microangiopathic hemolytic anemia, thrombocytopenia, renal failure, fluctuating neurologic symptoms, and what other feature?

(See answers next page.)

37. Reed-Sternberg cells

Blueprint Task: *Using Diagnostic and Laboratory Studies*
Cognitive Level: *Recall*

38. Penicillin

Children without a functioning spleen are at increased risk for severe infections due to encapsulated bacteria.
Blueprint Task: *Pharmaceutical Therapeutics*
Cognitive Level: *Analyze*

39. Pica

Blueprint Task: *History Taking and Performing Physical Examination*
Cognitive Level: *Recall*

40. Von Willebrand disease (VWD)

VWD is an inherited bleeding disorder that presents with spontaneous bruising, frequent mucous membrane bleeding, and menorrhagia.
Blueprint Task: *Formulating Most Likely Diagnosis*
Cognitive Level: *Apply*

41. Phlebotomy

The clinical vignette supports the diagnosis of polycythemia vera. The common history and physical findings outlined in the vignette are due to increased blood viscosity and volume.
Blueprint Task: *Clinical Intervention*
Cognitive Level: *Analyze*

42. Corticosteroids

Treatment of ITP (formerly termed idiopathic thrombocytopenic purpura) is dependent on risk of bleeding. Patients without active bleeding typically do not require pharmacologic therapy.
Blueprint Task: *Pharmaceutical Therapeutics*
Cognitive Level: *Apply*

43. Factor V Leiden mutation

Blueprint Task: *History Taking and Performing Physical Examination*
Cognitive Level: *Recall*

44. Immunoglobulin A (IgA) vasculitis

IgA vasculitis, formerly termed Henoch–Schönlein purpura, is the most common small-vessel vasculitis in children.
Blueprint Task: *Formulating Most Likely Diagnosis*
Cognitive Level: *Apply*

45. Fever

Blueprint Task: *History Taking and Performing Physical Examination*
Cognitive Level: *Recall*

46. A 67-year-old man who takes coumadin for chronic atrial fibrillation presents to the emergency department with recurrent epistaxis that is controlled with localized pressure. Laboratory studies reveal an INR of 12. After withholding warfarin, what is the next appropriate management step?

47. In a child with newly diagnosed aplastic anemia, what definitive treatment should be discussed with the family?

48. What type of thalassemia is characterized by severe dysfunction of two beta-globulin chains?

(See answers next page.)

46. Oral vitamin K

Warfarin interferes with the conversion cycle of vitamin K, disrupting the activity of coagulation factors II, VII, IX, and X. Thus, administration of vitamin K allows for new synthesis of coagulation factors. If clinically significant bleeding is present, then intravenous vitamin K may be necessary.

Blueprint Task: *Pharmaceutical Therapeutics*
Cognitive Level: *Apply*

47. Hematopoietic stem cell transplant

Blueprint Task: *Health Maintenance, Patient Education, and Preventive Measures*
Cognitive Level: *Recall*

48. Beta-thalassemia major

Blueprint Task: *Formulating Most Likely Diagnosis*
Cognitive Level: *Recall*

Infectious Diseases

1. What dermatologic reaction may occur in a patient with mononucleosis after taking amoxicillin?

2. What is the minimum induration size for a positive tuberculin skin test in a patient following an organ transplant?

3. A series of five vaccines protecting against diphtheria, tetanus, and acellular pertussis are routinely administered prior to the age of 7 years old. Following this series, a booster dose of what vaccine is recommended for adolescents 11–12 years old to provide further protection against these illnesses?

4. A 37-year-old man presents to the clinic with a red area near the armpit. Physical exam reveals a lesion located at the right mid-axillary line with a bright red outer border, target center, and partial central clearing. He recently returned from a hunting trip in the Northeastern region of the United States. What pharmacologic therapy is appropriate for the presumptive diagnosis?

5. A 22-year-old woman presents for her initial prenatal exam. During the routine screening, she is suspected of having gonorrhea. What is the most appropriate pharmacologic treatment regimen recommended for this patient?

6. What is the most common organism to cause ecthyma?

7. A 23-year-old man who is visiting Cameroon from the United States presents to the emergency department due to the sudden onset of large volume, explosive diarrhea over the last 24 hours. He describes the stool as hazy, without blood, and resembling "rice water." On physical exam, mucous membranes are dry with decreased skin turgor. What is the most important first step in the management of the presumptive diagnosis?

8. Pregnant women are advised to avoid changing a cat's litter box due to the risk of developing what dangerous infection?

(See answers next page.)

1. Morbilliform rash
Rash is a known feature associated with mononucleosis; however, if a patient with mononucleosis is exposed to antibiotics, such as amoxicillin, the likelihood of a rash developing increases significantly.
Blueprint Task: *History Taking and Performing Physical Examination*
Cognitive Level: *Apply*

2. 5 mm
An induration size of ≥ 5 mm is considered positive in patients with HIV, recent contact with active TB, fibrotic changes on a chest x-ray, organ transplant recipients, or otherwise immunosuppressed patients, as guided by the CDC.
Blueprint Task: *Using Diagnostic and Laboratory Studies*
Cognitive Level: *Apply*

3. TDap
Blueprint Task: *Health Maintenance, Patient Education, and Preventive Measures*
Cognitive Level: *Recall*

4. Doxycycline
The clinical vignette supports the diagnosis of Lyme disease caused by *Borrelia burgdorferi.*
Blueprint Task: *Clinical Intervention*
Cognitive Level: *Analyze*

5. Ceftriaxone 250 mg IM and azithromycin 1 g PO
Ceftriaxone is the preferred treatment for gonorrhea, and azithromycin is recommended for presumptive co-infection of chlamydia.
Blueprint Task: *Pharmaceutical Therapeutics*
Cognitive Level: *Apply*

6. *Streptococcus pyogenes*
Blueprint Task: *Applying Basic Scientific Concepts*
Cognitive Level: *Recall*

7. Fluid resuscitation
The clinical vignette supports the diagnosis of cholera. Hypovolemic shock is the leading cause of death in this condition, and the clinical vignette indicates hypovolemia.
Blueprint Task: *Clinical Intervention*
Cognitive Level: *Analyze*

8. Toxoplasmosis
Congenital toxoplasmosis infection may lead to spontaneous abortion, stillbirths, or other severe manifestations.
Blueprint Task: *Health Maintenance, Patient Education, and Preventive Measures*
Cognitive Level: *Apply*

9. A 28-year-old patient with AIDS presents to the clinic with visual blurring and floaters. The fundoscopic exam reveals retinal hemorrhages and edema. What laboratory test is required prior to an ophthalmologist referral to confirm the presumptive diagnosis?

10. The Systemic Inflammatory Response System (SIRS) criteria allocate one point each for specific features to include fever, tachycardia, leukocytosis, leukopenia, bandemia, and what other key physical exam finding?

11. A 9-year-old boy developed a sore throat 3 weeks ago but did not seek medical care. He now presents to the clinic with a fever of 38.9°C (102°F) and pink macules on the trunk. Musculoskeletal exam reveals pain, redness, and swelling of the right elbow and the left knee and ankle. He also has choreiform movements of the head and upper extremities. What is the most likely diagnosis?

12. What live-attenuated vaccine is contraindicated in a pediatric patient with a past history of intussusception?

13. A mother brings her 5-year-old daughter to the clinic for perianal pruritus, which is markedly worse at night. On physical exam, perianal excoriations are identified. What class of medication is most appropriate to treat the presumptive diagnosis?

14. What immunoglobulin responds first to an antigen?

15. A 24-year-old man presents with pruritic lesions to the foot and ankle after walking barefoot on the beach. What is the most likely diagnosis based on the following photo?

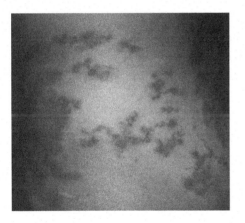

(*See answers next page.*)

9. No laboratory test is necessary

The clinical vignette supports the diagnosis of cytomegalovirus (CMV) retinitis, which is most often a clinical diagnosis based on history and characteristic retinal findings. Urgent referral to an ophthalmologist is necessary. Laboratory testing, such as PCR, is typically not utilized to determine diagnosis. While healthy patients with CMV infection are often asymptomatic, immunocompromised patients with CMV may develop complications such as retinitis or disseminated disease.

Blueprint Task: Using Diagnostic and Laboratory Studies
Cognitive Level: Analyze

10. Tachypnea

The SIRS criteria allow clinicians to recognize classic components of the physical exam and laboratory studies to diagnose sepsis. Early recognition and treatment are necessary due to the high mortality rate associated with sepsis and septic shock.

Blueprint Task: History Taking and Performing Physical Examination
Cognitive Level: Apply

11. Acute rheumatic fever

Jones criteria include major and minor criteria and are utilized when considering a diagnosis of acute rheumatic fever.

Blueprint Task: Formulating Most Likely Diagnosis
Cognitive Level: Apply

12. Rotavirus vaccine

Rotavirus is a common cause of severe gastrointestinal illness in infants and children. Intussusception is a serious gastrointestinal condition that causes telescoping of the intestines, which may lead to obstruction, ischemia, or infarction of the bowel.

Blueprint Task: Health Maintenance, Patient Education, and Preventive Measures
Cognitive Level: Apply

13. Anthelmintic

The clinical vignette supports the diagnosis of Enterobiasis, pinworms. Anti-parasitic drugs such as mebendazole or albendazole are recommended options.

Blueprint Task: Clinical Intervention
Cognitive Level: Analyze

14. IgM

Blueprint Task: Applying Basic Scientific Concepts
Cognitive Level: Recall

15. Cutaneous larva migrans (CLM)

CLM is the most common helminthic dermatosis. Travel history and exposure are important elements of the history.

Blueprint Task: Formulating Most Likely Diagnosis
Cognitive Level: Analyze

16. A 25-year-old man presents to the clinic with fatigue, headache, and paroxysms of chills, high fever, and sweats. He recently returned from a trip to Africa and experienced many mosquito bites. The patient did not utilize the recommended chemoprophylaxis. What laboratory test is recommended as the first line to screen for the presumptive diagnosis?

17. What does the H represent in the acronym TORCH?

18. A healthy 23-year-old patient presents to the clinic with a swollen, erythematous, tender bump on the arm. The patient is afebrile, otherwise asymptomatic, and without history of trauma or recurrent infection. Physical exam reveals a 1 cm tender, fluctuant, erythematous nodule on the right arm without lymphangitis or lymphadenopathy in the axillary or epitrochlear regions. What is the most appropriate clinical intervention for the presumptive diagnosis?

19. A 23-year-old woman presents to the clinic with frothy, yellow vaginal discharge for one week. She had unprotected sexual intercourse with a new partner 3 weeks ago. Wet mount shows motile organisms. What is the pathogen causing the presumptive diagnosis?

20. A 19-year-old man with incomplete immunization status presents to the clinic with a 4-day history of sore throat, hoarseness, rhinorrhea, cervical lymphadenopathy, and fever. Strep and mono screen are negative. Physical exam reveals a gray pseudomembrane that easily bleeds with manipulation. What is the most likely diagnosis?

21. A 21-year-old man presents to the clinic with a 5-day history of sore throat, headache, and myalgias. Physical exam reveals fever of 38.4°C (101.2°F) and cervical lymphadenopathy. He had unprotected intercourse 1 month ago. The strep and mono screens are negative. What initial laboratory test should be ordered to investigate the possibility of acute HIV syndrome?

22. What is the most common asymptomatic bacterial infectious disease reported in the United States?

23. What postexposure prophylaxis (PEP) for rabies is recommended following a high-risk animal bite?

(See answers next page.)

16. Thick and thin blood smear

The clinical vignette supports the diagnosis of malaria, caused by *Plasmodium* species. Thick and thin blood smear will evaluate for the presence of parasites. Chemoprophylaxis and other safety measures are recommended with travel to endemic areas.

Blueprint Task: Using Diagnostic and Laboratory Studies
Cognitive Level: Analyze

17. Herpes simplex virus

Blueprint Task: History Taking and Performing Physical Examination
Cognitive Level: Recall

18. Incision and drainage

The clinical vignette supports the diagnosis of localized abscess. Antibiotics are likely not necessary in this healthy patient. Oral antibiotics are typically used for recurrent or multiple abscesses or in patients with comorbidities or immunosuppression. Culture and susceptibility testing may be obtained as needed.

Blueprint Task: Clinical Intervention
Cognitive Level: Apply

19. *T. vaginalis*

The clinical vignette supports the diagnosis of trichomoniasis.

Blueprint Task: Formulating Most Likely Diagnosis
Cognitive Level: Analyze

20. Diphtheria

The physical exam describes the classic appearance of pharyngeal diphtheria. The diphtheric membrane is typically adherent and friable.

Blueprint Task: History Taking and Performing Physical Examination
Cognitive Level: Apply

21. HIV1/HIV2 combination antigen/antibody immunoassay

Acute HIV syndrome often resembles a viral illness and may develop within weeks of HIV infection. Acute HIV must remain in the differential, especially if risk factors are present.

Blueprint Task: Using Diagnostic and Laboratory Studies
Cognitive Level: Apply

22. *Chlamydia trachomatis*

Blueprint Task: Formulating Most Likely Diagnosis
Cognitive Level: Recall

23. Rabies immune globulin and rabies vaccine

There is no effective therapy for rabies. Wound care and PEP are essential.

Blueprint Task: Clinical Intervention
Cognitive Level: Apply

24. A 37-year-old woman with type 2 diabetes presents to the clinic with a 4-day history of vaginal pain, pruritus, and discharge described as whitish curds. She recently completed a course of antibiotics for sinusitis. What is the preferred oral treatment for the presumptive diagnosis?

25. What is the most common organism to cause a skin abscess in a healthy patient?

26. A 6-year-old girl presents to the clinic with a 3-day history of low-grade fever, upper respiratory symptoms, and sore throat. Yesterday, she developed vesicles on the palms and soles along with shallow erosions on the buccal mucosa and tongue. What is the presumptive diagnosis?

27. What is the most common source of atypical mycobacteria transmission?

28. A 52-year-old man presents to the emergency department with localized erythema and edema to the right arm. What bedside tool is helpful to differentiate between abscess and cellulitis?

29. A healthy 8-month-old child presents to the clinic for a visit in the month of October. Rotavirus, DTaP, Hib, IPV, and PCV13 immunizations were all given at 6 months of age. What additional immunization should be provided at today's visit?

30. A healthy 4-year-old boy presents with scant areas of honey-colored crusting around the nose and mouth. The patient is afebrile and playful. Parents are educated on skincare and proper hygiene. What pharmacologic therapy is recommended for the presumptive diagnosis?

31. A 91-year-old woman is admitted to the hospital due to rapidly progressive erysipelas. What bacteria is most commonly associated with this superficial skin infection?

32. A 9-month-old baby presents to the emergency department listless with droopy eyelids and has not been taking a bottle. Physical exam reveals ptosis, sluggish pupils, and hypotonia. Prior to symptom development, his mother began feeding the baby solids, which were canned at home. What is the presumptive diagnosis?

(*See answers next page.*)

24. Fluconazole

The clinical vignette supports a diagnosis of vulvovaginal candidiasis. Topical antifungals may also be beneficial for symptomatic relief.

Blueprint Task: Pharmaceutical Therapeutics
Cognitive Level: Analyze

25. *Staphylococcus aureus*

Blueprint Task: Applying Basic Scientific Concepts
Cognitive Level: Recall

26. Hand, foot and mouth disease (HFMD)

HFMD is a common viral exanthem in children under the age of 10, typically caused by coxsackievirus.

Blueprint Task: Formulating Most Likely Diagnosis
Cognitive Level: Apply

27. Environmental

Environmental sources, such as water and soil, frequently contribute to the development of atypical mycobacteria infection (*Mycobacterium* other than tuberculosis (MOTT)), which may affect any organ system.

Blueprint Task: History Taking and Performing Physical Examination
Cognitive Level: Apply

28. Point-of-care ultrasound (POCUS)

Blueprint Task: Using Diagnostic and Laboratory Studies
Cognitive Level: Recall

29. Influenza vaccine

During the first season of vaccination, children aged 6 months through 8 years require 2 doses of influenza vaccine $\geq$ 4 weeks apart.

Blueprint Task: Clinical Intervention
Cognitive Level: Apply

30. Topical antibiotic (mupirocin 2% ointment)

The clinical vignette supports the diagnosis of nonbullous impetigo. Topical antibiotics are recommended for limited eruptions.

Blueprint Task: Pharmaceutical Therapeutics
Cognitive Level: Analyze

31. Beta-hemolytic *Streptococci*

Blueprint Task: Applying Basic Scientific Concepts
Cognitive Level: Recall

32. Food-borne botulism

Improperly processed home-canned foods increase the risk of food-borne botulism.

Blueprint Task: Formulating Most Likely Diagnosis
Cognitive Level: Analyze

33. What is the first-line class of medication for the treatment of cutaneous larva migrans?

34. A 28-year-old man with a longstanding HIV recently experienced a 10-pound weight loss prompting the clinician to check a CD4 count, which was less than 200 cells/mcL. He developed a slowly progressive fever, nonproductive cough, and dyspnea over the last 7 days. Physical exam reveals faint bibasilar crackles, and chest radiograph demonstrates diffuse interstitial infiltrates. What is the first-line medication for the presumptive opportunistic infection?

35. What is the most common site for *Staphylococcus aureus* colonization?

36. A 54-year-old healthy, asymptomatic man presents to the clinic to discuss incidental findings on a chest radiograph. Radiographs reveal scattered calcifications of the lungs. He was born and raised along the Mississippi River. Based on this geographic location, what previous condition most likely caused the radiographic findings?

37. What is the classic description of the lesions associated with erythema multiforme that typically cause a rash on the face and extremities as seen in the following photo?

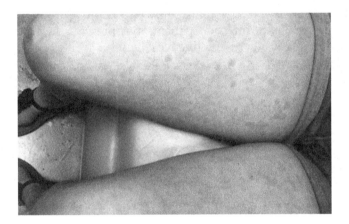

38. A 21-year-old woman presents to the clinic with a 7-day history of fatigue, myalgia, and sore throat. Physical exam reveals a low-grade fever, erythematous and enlarged tonsils with exudates, posterior cervical lymphadenopathy, and splenomegaly. What would be the characteristic finding on a complete blood count given the presumptive diagnosis?

39. Inactivated poliovirus (IPV) is routinely administered in the United States as a series of four shots prior to the age of 6 years old. At what age is the first IPV immunization typically administered?

40. A patient is found to be a carrier of methicillin-resistant *Staphylococcus aureus* (MRSA). In addition to chlorohexidine washes to prevent body colonization, what pharmacologic therapy is recommended to use intranasally?

41. A healthy, asymptomatic patient requires screening for tuberculosis. What diagnostic test is preferred if the patient is unable to follow up in 48 hours?

(See answers next page.)

33. Anthelmintic
Blueprint Task: *Clinical Intervention*
Cognitive Level: *Recall*

34. Trimethoprim sulfamethoxazole (TMP-SMZ)
The clinical vignette supports the diagnosis of *Pneumocystis jirovecii* pneumonia (PJP). The patient's risk for this opportunistic infection increases due to the development of AIDS, characterized by CD4 count <200 cells/mcL.
Blueprint Task: *Pharmaceutical Therapeutics*
Cognitive Level: *Analyze*

35. Anterior nares
Blueprint Task: *Applying Basic Scientific Concepts*
Cognitive Level: *Recall*

36. Histoplasmosis
Histoplasmosis is endemic in certain areas with high concentrations found in Ohio and along the Mississippi River. Inhalation of soil contaminated by bird and bat droppings is the vector for infection. In acute symptomatic infection, patients may present with features such as fever, malaise, myalgia, arthralgia, and nonproductive cough.
Blueprint Task: *Formulating Most Likely Diagnosis*
Cognitive Level: *Analyze*

37. Target lesions
Blueprint Task: *History Taking and Performing Physical Examination*
Cognitive Level: *Recall*

38. Lymphocytosis
The clinical vignette supports a diagnosis of infectious mononucleosis due to Epstein-Barr virus.
Blueprint Task: *Using Diagnostic and Laboratory Studies*
Cognitive Level: *Analyze*

39. 2 months old
Blueprint Task: *Health Maintenance, Patient Education, and Preventive Measures*
Cognitive Level: *Recall*

40. Mupirocin 2% ointment
MRSA colonization is associated with a significant increase risk of invasive MRSA infection, especially in hospitalized patients.
Blueprint Task: *Pharmaceutical Therapeutics*
Cognitive Level: *Apply*

41. Interferon-gamma release assay (IGRA)
Blueprint Task: *Clinical Intervention*
Cognitive Level: *Recall*

42. An 82-year-old man presented to the clinic one month ago with left-sided chest pain and hyperesthesia. The left chest revealed clusters of erythematous, vesicular eruptions over a single dermatome. Today, the patient returns to the clinic, reporting the rash resolved after 1 week, but he is still experiencing severe left-sided chest pain. What is the most likely complication associated with the initial presumptive diagnosis?

43. What is the characteristic primary lesion in a patient with *Treponema pallidum* infection?

44. Treatment is required in asymptomatic women with chlamydial and gonococcal infections to prevent what condition affecting the upper genital tract?

45. A 22-year-old woman presents to the clinic with multiple, well-defined papules and scattered flat lesions to the vulva and perianal skin. She had unprotected sex with multiple partners and has not received the HPV vaccine. What is the first-line class of medication recommended for the presumptive diagnosis?

46. A 14-year-old boy with incomplete immunizations presents to the clinic with a 4-day history of low-grade fever, body aches, headache, and decreased appetite. Physical exam reveals swelling and tenderness over both parotid glands. What is the presumptive diagnosis?

47. A 24-year-old woman presents to the clinic with a 4-day history of fever, cramping, abdominal pain, and 5–7 loose non-bloody stools daily. The two most common postinfectious sequalae associated with this condition are Guillain-Barré syndrome and reactive arthritis. What laboratory study confirms the presumptive diagnosis?

48. What is the most common birth defect affecting head size seen in newborns exposed to Zika virus in utero?

49. A 35-year-old man with a history of IV drug use presents to the emergency department with fever, cough, and pleuritic chest pain. Physical exam reveals 1–1.5 mm tender, purple-pink nodules with a pale center on the distal aspect of the digits. Echocardiogram is pending. What laboratory test is necessary to support the presumptive diagnosis?

50. Which formulation of the influenza vaccine is live-attenuated?

(See answers next page.)

42. Postherpetic neuralgia
The clinical vignette supports the diagnosis of herpes zoster infection. The most common complication is chronic neuropathic pain.
Blueprint Task: *Formulating Most Likely Diagnosis*
Cognitive Level: *Analyze*

43. Chancre
Treponema pallidum causes syphilis. A chancre is a painless papule or ulceration, commonly found on the genitalia.
Blueprint Task: *History Taking and Performing Physical Examination*
Cognitive Level: *Apply*

44. Pelvic inflammatory disease
Blueprint Task: *Health Maintenance, Patient Education, and Preventive Measures*
Cognitive Level: *Recall*

45. Topical immunomodulator
The clinical vignette supports anogenital warts caused by human papillomavirus. Topical application of podophyllotoxin or imiquimod is the primary pharmaceutical treatments. Other treatment options include cryotherapy, laser, or surgical interventions.
Blueprint Task: *Pharmaceutical Therapeutics*
Cognitive Level: *Analyze*

46. Mumps (paramyxovirus)
Parotitis is typically bilateral, and patients may describe pain with eating and speaking. Mumps may be associated with other rare complications such as orchitis.
Blueprint Task: *Formulating Most Likely Diagnosis*
Cognitive Level: *Apply*

47. Stool culture for *Campylobacter jejuni*
The clinical presentation and post-infectious sequelae are consistent with the diagnosis of *Campylobacter jejuni* infection.
Blueprint Task: *Using Diagnostic and Laboratory Studies*
Cognitive Level: *Apply*

48. Severe microcephaly
Blueprint Task: *History Taking and Performing Physical Examination*
Cognitive Level: *Recall*

49. Blood culture
The clinical vignette supports the diagnosis of bacterial endocarditis. The physical exam findings are consistent with Osler's nodes. A positive echocardiogram along with bacteremia via multiple blood cultures aids in the diagnosis of this condition.
Blueprint Task: *Using Diagnostic and Laboratory Studies*
Cognitive Level: *Analyze*

50. Intranasal
Blueprint Task: *Health Maintenance, Patient Education, and Preventive Measures*
Cognitive Level: *Recall*

51. A 42-year-old man presents to the clinic with a 3-day history of fever, headache, myalgias, and a rash that appeared yesterday on his ankles and is now spreading. He returned from a camping trip days before symptom onset. Physical exam reveals a macular, petechial rash over the wrists, ankles, palms, soles, and trunk. What is the pharmacologic treatment of choice for the presumptive diagnosis?

52. A 33-year-old man with AIDS presents to the clinic with progressive dysphagia and odynophagia. Endoscopy reveals white plaques with underlying friable mucosa. KOH stain demonstrates hyphae. What is the presumptive diagnosis?

53. What term defines the classic dermatologic presentation of stage 1 infection from *Borrelia burgdorferi?*

54. A 19-year-old woman is diagnosed with pelvic inflammatory disease. She is treated for gonorrhea and chlamydia while sexually transmitted infection (STI) testing is pending and is advised that her current partner should be evaluated and treated. What primary education should be provided to this patient who is sexually active to decrease future risk of STI?

55. What are the four first-line pharmacologic agents for the treatment of active tuberculosis?

56. A 56-year-old woman recently returned from a vacation to Arizona. She enjoyed golfing and riding ATVs in the desert. Since returning home, she developed a cough, pleuritic chest pain, fatigue, night sweats, and diffuse arthralgias. On physical exam, painful erythematous nodules are present on the lower legs. Radiographs reveal a pulmonary infiltrate in the right upper lobe and hilar adenopathy. What is the presumptive diagnosis?

57. A 9-month-old infant presents to the clinic with a 2-day history of fever reaching 34.4°C (103°F). The baby has been active with mild irritability, and the physical exam reveals no abnormalities. The clinician predicts the fever will likely abate in the next 24 hours and a rash will appear. Given the presumptive diagnosis, what is the most likely description of the anticipated rash?

58. What is the most common organism causing infection from a cat bite?

(See answers next page.)

51. Doxycycline

The clinical vignette supports the diagnosis of Rocky Mountain spotted fever, a potentially fatal illness caused by *Rickettsia rickettsii*.

Blueprint Task: *Pharmaceutical Therapeutics*
Cognitive Level: *Analyze*

52. Esophageal candidiasis

Esophageal candidiasis is more common in immunocompromised patients, and fluconazole is the treatment of choice.

Blueprint Task: *Formulating Most Likely Diagnosis*
Cognitive Level: *Analyze*

53. Erythema migrans

Borrelia burgdorferi is the causative agent of Lyme disease. A bull's eye rash appears around site of the tick bite typically within a week. Viral-like illness with myalgias, headache, and fever are also common.

Blueprint Task: *History Taking and Performing Physical Examination*
Cognitive Level: *Analyze*

54. Advise use of barrier contraceptive

Blueprint Task: *Health Maintenance, Patient Education, and Preventive Measures*
Cognitive Level: *Recall*

55. Isoniazid, rifampin, pyrazinamide, ethambutol

Treatment usually consists of utilizing all four medications for 2 months, followed by isoniazid and rifampin for the next 4 months.

Blueprint Task: *Pharmaceutical Therapeutics*
Cognitive Level: *Apply*

56. Primary pulmonary coccidioidomycosis

Acute presentation of coccidioidomycosis (Valley fever) should be suspected based on recent travel to an endemic region, exposure to contaminated soil, pulmonary and extrapulmonary manifestations, and imaging findings.

Blueprint Task: *Formulating Most Likely Diagnosis*
Cognitive Level: *Analyze*

57. Erythematous macular or maculopapular eruptions

The clinical vignette supports the diagnosis of roseola infantum. Rash is typically found on neck, trunk, and buttocks, and resolves within 48 hours.

Blueprint Task: *History Taking and Performing Physical Examination*
Cognitive Level: *Analyze*

58. *Pasteurella multocida*

Blueprint Task: *Applying Basic Scientific Concepts*
Cognitive Level: *Recall*

Musculoskeletal System

1. What is the provocative maneuver for developmental dysplasia of the hip that is performed by attempting to displace the femoral head posteriorly while the hip is maintained in flexion and adduction?

2. What is the best imaging study to evaluate for a suspected labral tear in the shoulder?

3. A 63-year-old man presents with ongoing low back pain. Pain worsens with extension and is relieved with lying down or leaning over, such as when pushing a shopping cart. He also has progressive bilateral leg pain that worsens with walking or standing and is relieved with sitting. What is the most likely diagnosis?

4. The parents of a 2-year-old girl report they have noticed that the toddler seems to limp every morning for weeks but then improves through the day. Less than five joints are involved, and no other symptoms are present. The patient was referred to rheumatology and physical therapy. What additional referral is necessary to prevent a serious complication of this type of juvenile idiopathic arthritis?

5. A 22-year-old woman presents with a mildly painful soft-tissue mass on the volar aspect of the right wrist. The mass fluctuates in size and is noticeably larger with activity. What treatment recommendation provides the lowest risk for recurrence?

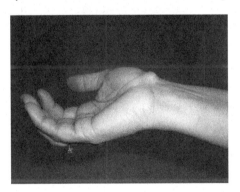

6. A pharmacologic antimalarial therapy is commonly prescribed for patients with systemic lupus erythematosus (SLE). What commonly used medication also warrants regular eye examinations for retinal changes?

7. Which nerve is most likely to be injured in an acute shoulder dislocation causing deltoid weakness and numbness over the skin of the upper arm?

8. A 15-year-old basketball player presents to the clinic with episodic bilateral knee pain worsening over the last few weeks with the start of the new basketball season. He denies trauma and states the pain is worse on the left. On physical exam, point tenderness is noted bilaterally over the tibial tuberosity. What is the most likely diagnosis?

1. Barlow

Barlow and Ortolani tests are both key physical exam techniques for developmental dysplasia of the hip. Barlow test is not beneficial in infants with a dislocated hip at rest, but Ortolani test can still be attempted to assess ability to reduce the hip.

Blueprint Task: History Taking and Performing Physical Examination
Cognitive Level: Apply

2. MR arthrogram

Blueprint Task: Using Diagnostic and Laboratory Studies
Cognitive Level: Recall

3. Spinal stenosis

Spinal stenosis commonly produces pain with extension and neurogenic claudication that improves with sitting, lying down, or bending forward.

Blueprint Task: Formulating Most Likely Diagnosis
Cognitive Level: Apply

4. Ophthalmology

The clinical vignette supports the diagnosis of oligoarthritis in which iritis or uveitis can occur. Interval surveillance is necessary to avoid permanent vision loss.

Blueprint Task: Health Maintenance, Patient Education, and Preventive Measures
Cognitive Level: Analyze

5. Surgical excision

The clinical vignette supports the diagnosis of ganglion cyst. Conservative treatment of a ganglion cyst includes observation, NSAIDs, and/or bracing for pain control. If pain continues, aspiration both with or without a corticosteroid injection or surgical intervention is appropriate. Regardless of intervention, recurrence is common.

Blueprint Task: Clinical Intervention
Cognitive Level: Analyze

6. Hydroxychloroquine

Hydroxychloroquine decreases severity and frequency of SLE exacerbations and prolongs survival.

Blueprint Task: Pharmaceutical Therapeutics
Cognitive Level: Apply

7. Axillary

Blueprint Task: Applying Basic Scientific Concepts
Cognitive Level: Recall

8. Osgood-Schlatter disease

Osgood-Schlatter disease is a pediatric condition caused by apophysitis of the tibial tubercle.

Blueprint Task: Formulating Most Likely Diagnosis
Cognitive Level: Apply

9. A 68-year-old man with a history of hypertension, type 2 diabetes, and BMI of 32 kg/ m$_2$ presents with severe pain, erythema, and edema at the base of his left, first toe that developed overnight. The bedsheets exacerbate his pain. He consumed an increased amount of red meat and alcohol. What would be the expected crystal analysis findings on arthrocentesis based on the presumptive diagnosis?

10. The McMurray test is a specialized physical exam technique used to evaluate for an injury to what anatomic structure?

11. A 34-year-old man presents to the clinic with severe pain in the distal aspect of his right index finger after dropping a 10-pound weight on the finger today. He has full range of motion, strength, and sensation intact. The nail bed reveals a collection of blood visible under a large portion of the nail. Radiographs reveal no fracture. What is the recommended intervention for pain relief?

12. What is the most common serious side effect from chronic use of nonsteroidal anti-inflammatories (NSAIDs)?

13. Urgent intervention with antibiotics, irrigation, and debridement is required for open fractures to prevent what bone condition?

14. What term describes a burst fracture of the atlas identified with an open-mouth odontoid view radiograph?

15. A 5-year-old girl fell from the monkey bars onto her outstretched hand with the elbow in hyperextension. She presents to the clinic with left elbow swelling and pain localized to the distal humerus. The anterior humeral line does not intersect the capitellum on radiographs consistent with a displaced supracondylar fracture. What physical exam technique will assess for the most likely neuropraxia associated with this injury?

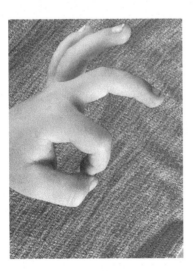

16. What is the most specific laboratory blood test for rheumatoid arthritis?

17. A 23-year-old man presents with localized, dull achy pain to the right proximal femoral shaft. The bone pain awakens him at night but is relieved with NSAIDs. What benign tumor classically presents with these historical findings?

(See answers next page.)

9. Needle-shaped, negatively birefringent monosodium urate crystals

The clinical vignette supports the diagnosis of gout. Joint aspirate reveals characteristic crystals, most commonly deposited in the first metatarsal phalangeal joint.

Blueprint Task: Using Diagnostic and Laboratory Studies

Cognitive Level: Analyze

10. Meniscus

Blueprint Task: History Taking and Performing Physical Examination

Cognitive Level: Recall

11. Trephination

The clinical vignette supports a subungual hematoma. Trephination of the nail is recommended to relieve pain and allow drainage. Tools used include a nail drill, needle, or electrocautery.

Blueprint Task: Clinical Intervention

Cognitive Level: Analyze

12. Gastrointestinal toxicity

Blueprint Task: Pharmaceutical Therapeutics

Cognitive Level: Recall

13. Osteomyelitis

Open fractures significantly increase the risk of local microbial spread and may lead to bone infection.

Blueprint Task: Health Maintenance, Patient Education, and Preventive Measures

Cognitive Level: Apply

14. Jefferson fracture

Blueprint Task: Formulating Most Likely Diagnosis

Cognitive Level: Recall

15. "OK" sign

Supracondylar fractures are most likely to cause trauma to the anterior interosseus nerve (AIN). AIN is a motor branch of the median nerve and innervates flexor digitorum profundus of the index finger and flexor pollicus longus allowing for interphalangeal (IP) flexion of the thumb and distal interphalangeal (DIP) flexion of the index finger.

Blueprint Task: History Taking and Performing Physical Examination

Cognitive Level: Analyze

16. Anti-CCP antibodies

Blueprint Task: Using Diagnostic and Laboratory Studies

Cognitive Level: Recall

17. Osteoid osteoma

Osteoid osteomas are benign osteoid-forming tumors. Pain is related to high concentrations of prostaglandins released from the center of the tumor (nidus) and is relieved by NSAIDs.

Blueprint Task: Formulating Most Likely Diagnosis

Cognitive Level: Apply

18. Waddell signs are used in the evaluation of what condition?

19. A 53-year-old man with type 2 diabetes presents for ongoing catching and occasional locking of the right thumb. On physical exam, thumb is in flexion at rest and must be forced to return to extension. A tender nodule is palpated on the palmar aspect of the hand. The patient reports previous injections in the thumb, but symptoms continue to return. What is the definitive treatment for this condition?

20. Which class of medication is beneficial in the management of osteogenesis imperfecta by improving bone density and decreasing the risk of fractures?

21. A 17-year-old soccer player presents to the emergency department for a tibial shaft fracture he sustained after being kicked in the lower leg 2 hours ago. The clinician avoids immediate casting for initial treatment to prevent what condition?

22. A 29-year-old man presents with ongoing low back pain that is worse in the mornings. He denies trauma. On physical exam, decreased active and passive lumbar flexion is noted with associated pain. Plain radiographs of the spine and pelvis reveal fusion of the sacroiliac joints. What is the most helpful laboratory test to support your presumptive diagnosis?

23. What specialized physical exam assesses knee stability following an anterior cruciate ligament injury by translating the tibia anteriorly on the femur with slight knee flexion with the patient supine?

24. A 55-year-old woman presents to the clinic with progressive difficulty getting up from a chair and climbing stairs for months. Physical exam reveals symmetric proximal muscle weakness, erythema of the shoulders consistent with shawl sign, and violaceous discoloration around the eyes consistent with heliotrope rash. She has an elevated creatinine kinase and aldolase. What is the most likely diagnosis?

25. What is the common congenital chest wall abnormality presenting as a sunken appearance of the anterior thoracic wall?

(*See answers next page.*)

18. Low back pain
Blueprint Task: Health Maintenance, Patient Education, and Preventive Measures
Cognitive Level: *Recall*

19. Surgical release of the A1 pulley
Stenosing tenosynovitis (trigger thumb or finger) typically responds well to steroid injections of the flexor tendon sheath. Surgical intervention is indicated with fixed locking or recurring symptoms. Repeat steroid injections may lead to tendon degeneration and rupture.
Blueprint Task: Clinical Intervention
Cognitive Level: *Analyze*

20. Bisphosphonate
Blueprint Task: Pharmaceutical Therapeutics
Cognitive Level: *Recall*

21. Compartment syndrome
Compartment syndrome may result from increasing pressure within a limited space, causing compression to anatomic structures including nerves and vessels. Casting too early increases the risk of compartment syndrome by restricting the space for swelling caused by the injury.
Blueprint Task: Health Maintenance, Patient Education, and Preventive Measures
Cognitive Level: *Apply*

22. HLA-B27
The genetic marker, HLA-B27, is highly suggestive of ankylosing spondylitis.
Blueprint Task: Using Diagnostic and Laboratory Studies
Cognitive Level: *Analyze*

23. Lachman test
Blueprint Task: History Taking and Performing Physical Examination
Cognitive Level: *Recall*

24. Dermatomyositis
Patients with dermatomyositis typically present with proximal muscle weakness found in polymyositis but also have classic dermatologic manifestations such as shawl sign, heliotrope rash, and Gottron papules.
Blueprint Task: Formulating Most Likely Diagnosis
Cognitive Level: *Apply*

25. Pectus excavatum
Blueprint Task: Formulating Most Likely Diagnosis
Cognitive Level: *Recall*

26. A father presents to the clinic with his 2-year-old daughter after playing airplane in the backyard. He describes swinging her in a circle while holding onto her wrists when he felt a popping sensation in the right arm. She is guarding and refusing to use the arm. What is the most appropriate management?

27. A 24-year-old woman presents with left-sided low back pain that radiates down the lateral aspect of her left thigh. Physical exam reveals weakness of the tibialis anterior and numbness of the great toe on the left. Lumbar MRI indicates a herniated disc. At what level would herniation be most likely based on her symptoms?

28. A healthy 72-year-old man presents to the clinic with longstanding bilateral knee and hand pain that improves with rest. Upon waking, he feels mild stiffness that lasts for less than 20 minutes. He has no systemic symptoms. Radiographs of the knees reveal narrowed joint space and osteophytes. What is the initial class of medication recommended for the presumptive diagnosis?

29. Which of the six Ps is the earliest sign of compartment syndrome on physical exam?

30. What criteria are used when determining if a patient requires radiographic imaging following an ankle injury?

31. A 6-year-old boy is brought to the clinic by his parents because of an atraumatic limp that has developed over the last few weeks. He describes mild pain in the groin and thigh following activity. Physical exam reveals limited abduction and internal rotation on the right. Anteroposterior pelvic radiographs reveal flattening of the femoral epiphysis on the right. What is the most likely diagnosis?

32. What term describes an abnormal anterior fat pad on radiographs suggestive of an occult elbow fracture?

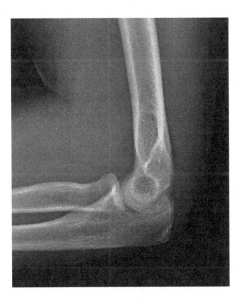

(*See answers next page.*)

26. Radial head reduction

The clinical scenario is consistent with a nursemaid's elbow. Either supination followed by elbow flexion or hyperpronation are therapeutic maneuvers to reduce a radial head subluxation. Radiographs are not typically warranted.

Blueprint Task: *Clinical Intervention*

Cognitive Level: *Analyze*

27. L4-L5

The clinical vignette supports the diagnosis of lumbar radiculopathy with dermatomal findings consistent with an L5 nerve root impingement.

Blueprint Task: *Applying Basic Scientific Concepts*

Cognitive Level: *Apply*

28. Nonsteroidal anti-inflammatories (NSAIDs)

The clinical vignette supports the diagnosis of osteoarthritis. Topical and oral NSAIDs may be beneficial for symptomatic osteoarthritis.

Blueprint Task: *Pharmaceutical Therapeutics*

Cognitive Level: *Analyze*

29. Pain

Aggravation of pain with active or passive stretching of muscles within a compartment may be the only finding on physical exam, and it is the most sensitive test for the evaluation of compartment syndrome. Pallor, paresthesia, poikilothermia, paralysis, and pulselessness are later findings associated with compartment syndrome.

Blueprint Task: *History Taking and Performing Physical Examination*

Cognitive Level: *Analyze*

30. Ottawa ankle rules

Blueprint Task: *Health Maintenance, Patient Education, and Preventive Measures*

Cognitive Level: *Recall*

31. Legg-Calve-Perthes disease (Perthes disease)

Perthes disease is idiopathic osteonecrosis of the proximal femoral epiphysis.

Blueprint Task: *Formulating Most Likely Diagnosis*

Cognitive Level: *Apply*

32. Sail sign

Abnormal fat pad on radiographs may indicate a traumatic hemarthrosis associated with a fracture. The anterior fat pad is commonly referred to as a sail sign based on the appearance on imaging.

Blueprint Task: *Using Diagnostic and Laboratory Studies*

Cognitive Level: *Apply*

33. A 35-year-old woman with a history of anxiety presents with chronic diffuse myalgias for 6 months. The patient reports fatigue, headaches, and cognitive difficulties. Physical exam reveals multiple muscular tender points and is otherwise unremarkable. What are the expected lab findings based on the presumptive diagnosis?

34. A 2-year-old girl caught her foot on the side of the slide while riding down on the lap of her older sibling. She displayed immediate pain and continues to refuse to bear weight on the affected limb. What term is commonly used to describe this type of fracture?

35. What is the largest sesamoid in the body?

36. A 43-year-old woman recently diagnosed with polymyositis is experiencing progressive symmetric proximal muscle weakness. What is the first-line pharmacologic therapy?

37. What condition is triggered by gastrointestinal or genitourinary infections and is commonly associated with inflammatory arthritis, conjunctivitis, uveitis, and urethritis?

38. A child presents with an intermittent macular salmon-colored rash, diffuse lymphadenopathy, and arthralgias in the wrists, knees, and ankles. History reveals recurrent spiking fevers >38.5°C (101.3°F) that resolve through the day. In the absence of infection or malignancy, what would be the expected findings on complete blood count?

39. A 35-year-old man sustained a forearm injury with direct impact to the proximal ulna. Radiographs reveal a transverse fracture of the ulna with an associated radial head dislocation. What term describes this type of injury?

40. A 50-year-old man presents to the emergency department with worsening pain and swelling of the left olecranon with warmth and redness over the last 48 hours. He developed a fever of 38.3°C (101°F) this morning. What intervention is both diagnostic and therapeutic?

(*See answers next page.*)

33. Normal laboratory studies

The clinical vignette supports the diagnosis of fibromyalgia. The hallmark of diagnosis is widespread body pain lasting at least 3 months. Laboratory tests are beneficial to assess for other etiologies.

Blueprint Task: *Using Diagnostic and Laboratory Studies*
Cognitive Level: *Analyze*

34. Toddler fracture

Toddler fracture is a spiral fracture to the distal tibia caused by a twisting mechanism. This diagnosis is often missed or delayed due to presumed injury to the ankle or foot in a young child limping. The mechanism of injury and age of the patient should prompt evaluation of the tibia for injury.

Blueprint Task: *Formulating Most Likely Diagnosis*
Cognitive Level: *Analyze*

35. Patella

Blueprint Task: *Applying Basic Scientific Concepts*
Cognitive Level: *Recall*

36. Glucocorticoids

Blueprint Task: *Pharmaceutical Therapeutics*
Cognitive Level: *Recall*

37. Reactive arthritis

Reactive arthritis (formerly termed Reiter syndrome) is typically precipitated by dysentery or sexually transmitted infections. Oligoarthritis often affects the lower extremities and is frequently associated with enthesitis and extra-articular manifestations.

Blueprint Task: *Formulating Most Likely Diagnosis*
Cognitive Level: *Apply*

38. Leukocytosis and reactive thrombocytosis

The clinical vignette supports the diagnosis of systemic juvenile idiopathic arthritis. Additional lab findings may include elevated ESR and CRP with a negative ANA and RF.

Blueprint Task: *Using Diagnostic and Laboratory Studies*
Cognitive Level: *Analyze*

39. Monteggia fracture dislocation

Blueprint Task: *Using Diagnostic and Laboratory Studies*
Cognitive Level: *Recall*

40. Bursal aspiration

The clinical vignette supports the diagnosis of septic olecranon bursitis. Bursal fluid analysis and culture are recommended along with antibiotics.

Blueprint Task: *Clinical Intervention*
Cognitive Level: *Analyze*

41. What class of medication is the first line in the management of Raynaud's phenomenon?

42. A 64-year-old man presents with months of fatigue, intermittent low-grade fever, and diffuse arthralgias and myalgias. Skin exam demonstrates livedo reticularis and ulcers of the lower extremities. Laboratory workup reveals elevated ESR, CRP, creatinine, AST, and ALT. Urinalysis is positive for proteinuria and hematuria. Antineutrophil cytoplasmic antibodies (ANCA) are negative. Polyarteritis nodosa (PAN) is suspected. What infection is most commonly linked to this diagnosis?

43. Which three primary cancer sites most commonly metastasize to the bone?

44. A 51-year-old woman presents to the clinic with chronic joint pain in the fingers, wrists, and knees and morning stiffness. Physical exam reveals ulnar deviation of the metacarpophalangeal joints with erythema, edema, and tenderness of the proximal interphalangeal joints. Radiographs of the hands demonstrate juxta-articular demineralization. What is the presumptive diagnosis?

45. The clinician asks the patient to grasp the thumb into a closed fist followed by ulnar deviation. Pain along the dorsoradial aspect of the wrist with this maneuver is suggestive of what condition?

46. An 81-year-old woman with hyperparathyroidism reports recurrent flares of knee pain, erythema, and edema. Crystal analysis on arthrocentesis of the knee reveals weakly positively birefringent, rhomboid-shaped calcium pyrophosphate crystals. What is the most likely diagnosis?

47. A 16-year-old competitive gymnast presents with midline low back pain that is aggravated by extension. She denies recent trauma. Physical exam reveals point tenderness to palpation at L5, hamstring tightness, and pain with single-leg hyperextension. Radiographs of the lumbar spine reveal a "Scottie dog" sign at L5. What is the most likely diagnosis?

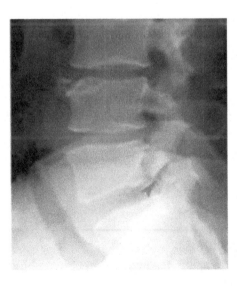

48. What is the most common position of the lower extremity following a hip dislocation?

(See answers next page.)

41. Calcium channel blockers

Blueprint Task: Pharmaceutical Therapeutics
Cognitive Level: Recall

42. Hepatitis B virus

Polyarteritis nodosa (PAN) is a systemic necrotizing vasculitis that may affect any organ. However, unlike other forms of vasculitis, PAN is not associated with the presence of ANCA.

Blueprint Task: Applying Basic Scientific Concepts
Cognitive Level: Apply

43. Lung, Breast, Prostate

Blueprint Task: Health Maintenance, Patient Education, and Preventive Measures
Cognitive Level: Recall

44. Rheumatoid arthritis

Rheumatoid arthritis is a chronic systemic disease characterized by inflammatory arthritis with extended morning stiffness. Another potential finding includes nodules on the dorsal surface of the forearm.

Blueprint Task: Formulating Most Likely Diagnosis
Cognitive Level: Apply

45. De Quervain's tenosynovitis

Finkelstein test is positive for de Quervain's if the maneuver aggravates pain along the tendons of the first dorsal compartment.

Blueprint Task: History Taking and Performing Physical Examination
Cognitive Level: Apply

46. Calcium pyrophosphate crystal deposition (CPPD) disease

CPPD, also called as pseudogout, is most commonly found in the knee.

Blueprint Task: Using Diagnostic and Laboratory Studies
Cognitive Level: Apply

47. Spondylolysis

The incidence of pars interarticularis fracture is increased in athletes engaged in activities in which there is repetitive flexion/extension and rotational movements. The Scottie dog sign reflects a fracture of the pars interarticularis and appears like a collar around the neck of the Scottie dog consistent with spondylolysis.

Blueprint Task: Formulating Most Likely Diagnosis
Cognitive Level: Analyze

48. Shortened with adduction and internal rotation

The majority of hip dislocations are posterior. The classic presentation of the leg is critical to differentiate from a femoral neck fracture and indicates the need for emergent reduction.

Blueprint Task: History Taking and Performing Physical Examination
Cognitive Level: Apply

49. What is the most common Salter-Harris classification type, which involves the metaphysis and the physis in a pediatric fracture?

50. A 36-year-old woman presents to the clinic with increasing pain in the lateral aspect of the hip, which is exacerbated when rolling on her side at night. Localized tenderness is noted over the greater trochanter. Radiographs are unremarkable. She has been working with a physical therapist, applying ice during exacerbations, and increasing NSAID dosing to control pain. What is the next step in her treatment?

51. What is the best study for the evaluation of osteoporosis in postmenopausal women following a fragility fracture?

52. A 24-year-old woman with a strong family history of autoimmune disorders presents with progressive fatigue, discoloration of the fingers with exposure to cold, heartburn, and occasional dysphagia with solid foods. Physical exam reveals calcium deposits under the skin and telangiectasias. The skin of the hands appears tight and thickened. What is the presumptive diagnosis?

53. A 53-year-old man presents to the clinic with an insidious onset of left anterolateral shoulder pain. He complains of a dull ache in his shoulder that disrupts sleep. On physical exam, the pain is worsened by internally rotating the shoulder with the palm down while maintaining the shoulder and elbow in 90 degrees of flexion. What specialized physical exam test does this technique describe?

54. A 22-year-old man sustained a traumatic injury to the right wrist earlier today. Pain is localized radially with point tenderness over the snuffbox. Radiographs are negative for fracture. What clinical intervention is warranted at this appointment?

55. What class of medication is first-line management for polymyalgia rheumatica?

56. What is the primary difference between rickets and osteomalacia?

(See answers next page.)

49. Type II
Blueprint Task: Applying Basic Scientific Concepts
Cognitive Level: Recall

50. Corticosteroid injection
The clinical vignette supports the diagnosis of greater trochanteric pain syndrome. Corticosteroid injections can be diagnostic and therapeutic.
Blueprint Task: Clinical Intervention
Cognitive Level: Analyze

51. Dual-energy x-ray absorptiometry (DXA)
Blueprint Task: Health Maintenance, Patient Education, and Preventive Measures
Cognitive Level: Recall

52. Systemic sclerosis
The clinical vignette supports the diagnosis of limited cutaneous systemic sclerosis (CREST syndrome), the most common form of systemic sclerosis. Elements of CREST include calcinosis, Raynaud's phenomenon, esophageal dysfunction, sclerodactyly, and telangiectasias.
Blueprint Task: Formulating Most Likely Diagnosis
Cognitive Level: Apply

53. Hawkins impingement test
Hawkins impingement test evaluates for underlying subacromial impingement syndrome. Chronic narrowing of the space between the proximal humerus and the distal acromion is commonly due to repetitive mechanical trauma or overuse.
Blueprint Task: History Taking and Performing Physical Examination
Cognitive Level: Apply

54. Thumb spica splint immobilization
The clinical vignette supports a presumptive diagnosis of a scaphoid fracture. Radiographic evidence of the fracture may be delayed, and treatment should be provided based on clinical suspicion due to the risk of avascular necrosis. Follow-up imaging is indicated.
Blueprint Task: Clinical Intervention
Cognitive Level: Analyze

55. Corticosteroids
Blueprint Task: Pharmaceutical Therapeutics
Cognitive Level: Recall

56. Skeletal maturity
Both conditions involve impaired bone mineralization primarily due to vitamin D deficiency. Rickets occurs in the skeletally immature prior to physeal closure and osteomalacia occurs following physeal closure.
Blueprint Task: Applying Basic Scientific Concepts
Cognitive Level: Apply

57. During a routine well-child check for a newborn, the chin appears rotated to the right with the head tilted to the left at rest. Mild plagiocephaly is noted. What is the initial management recommendation?

58. What common musculoskeletal management recommendation for upper extremity conditions increases the risk of developing adhesive capsulitis?

59. What condition produces an exaggerated forward flexion curvature of the upper spine and is best identified during physical examination from the side?

60. An 11-year-old boy presents with increasing left anterior hip pain. He is febrile and unable to weight-bear on the left lower extremity. At rest, he prefers to maintain hip flexion and abduction. What criteria will guide the need for hip aspiration and help to differentiate from transient synovitis in a pediatric patient?

61. What is the term for hyperextension at the proximal interphalangeal joint and flexion at the distal interphalangeal joint?

62. What class of medication should be initiated once rheumatoid arthritis is confirmed to preserve function, minimize pain, and decrease inflammation?

63. A 56-year-old woman sustained a high-energy trauma to the chest wall. Physical exam reveals paradoxical respirations. What is the minimum number of fractured ribs to cause this unstable condition?

64. A 20-year-old basketball player reports a sudden severe pain described as a "gunshot to the back of the leg" with an audible pop. He was rapidly changing direction while running when the injury occurred. While the patient is prone, the clinician squeezes the calf, examining for plantar flexion. What specialized physical exam test is being performed?

(See answers next page.)

57. Passive stretching

The clinical vignette supports the diagnosis of congenital torticollis with tightening of the left sternocleidomastoid. Passive stretching is an effective treatment option, often guided by physical therapy.

Blueprint Task: Clinical Intervention

Cognitive Level: Analyze

58. Shoulder immobilization

Prolonged shoulder immobilization for conditions including fractures, dislocations, surgery, or soft tissue injuries should be avoided. When immobilization is necessary, minimizing the length of time and introducing early motion of the shoulder will help to prevent adhesive capsulitis (also known as frozen shoulder).

Blueprint Task: Health Maintenance, Patient Education, and Preventive Measures

Cognitive Level: Apply

59. Hyperkyphosis

Blueprint Task: Formulating Most Likely Diagnosis

Cognitive Level: Recall

60. Kocher criteria

The clinical scenario is worrisome for acute septic arthritis of the left hip. The Kocher criteria includes fever >38.5°C (101.3°F), non-weight bearing, elevated WBC >12,000 cells/mm^3, and elevated ESR >40 mm/hr. Elevated CRP is an independent risk factor for septic arthritis. MRI of the hip is also helpful in determining the diagnosis.

Blueprint Task: Using Diagnostic and Laboratory Studies

Cognitive Level: Analyze

61. Swan neck deformity

Blueprint Task: History Taking and Performing Physical Examination

Cognitive Level: Recall

62. Disease-modifying antirheumatic drugs (DMARDs)

Blueprint Task: Pharmaceutical Therapeutics

Cognitive Level: *Recall*

63. Three or more adjacent ribs with segmental fractures

The clinical vignette supports the diagnosis of flail chest.

Blueprint Task: Applying Basic Scientific Concepts

Cognitive Level: Analyze

64. Thompson test

The clinical vignette supports the diagnosis of an Achilles tendon rupture. The Thompson test is positive if squeezing the calf does not elicit plantar flexion.

Blueprint Task: History Taking and Performing Physical Examination

Cognitive Level: Analyze

65. A 35-year-old man tripped on a curb with direct impact to the knee. He was immediately unable to extend the knee and has a large knee effusion. Tenderness is localized to the patella. In what position should the patient be immobilized?

66. What class of medication is associated with the potential complication of osteonecrosis of the jaw?

67. A 43-year-old secretary presents to the clinic with worsening pain and numbness in her fingers that exacerbates at night and with typing. Physical exam reveals atrophy of the thenar eminence. Tapping the volar aspect of the wrist causes shooting pain and numbness along the median nerve distribution. What specialized test is being performed?

68. What acromioclavicular (AC) joint injury classification describes an AC ligament tear with a coracoclavicular ligament sprain?

69. A 64-year-old man presents to the clinic for a follow-up of gout. Over the past year, he has experienced four flares managed with ibuprofen. What medication is most commonly prescribed for prevention of acute exacerbations and chronic manifestation?

70. What surgical emergency must be considered in a patient with saddle anesthesia?

71. A 13-year-old athlete sustained an ankle injury during a football game 2 days ago. Radiographs reveal a complex Salter-Harris (SH) IV fracture of the tibia. What term describes this type of fracture in an adolescent patient?

72. A 10-year-old premenarchal girl presents for follow-up of asymptomatic adolescent idiopathic scoliosis. Radiographs reveal a thoracolumbar curvature with a Cobb angle of 35°. What treatment is recommended?

(*See answers next page.*)

65. Full extension

The clinical vignette supports the diagnosis of a patellar fracture. Full knee extension may be provided with a long-leg splint, knee immobilizer, or hinged knee brace locked in extension.

Blueprint Task: Clinical Intervention

Cognitive Level: Analyze

66. Bisphosphonates

Blueprint Task: Pharmaceutical Therapeutics

Cognitive Level: Recall

67. Tinel test

The clinical vignette supports the diagnosis of carpal tunnel syndrome (CTS). Conditions such as rheumatoid arthritis, hypothyroidism, and pregnancy may increase the risk of developing CTS.

Blueprint Task: History Taking and Performing Physical Examination

Cognitive Level: Analyze

68. Type II

Blueprint Task: Applying Basic Scientific Concepts

Cognitive Level: Recall

69. Allopurinol

Allopurinol is a xanthine oxidase inhibitor and is not typically initiated during an acute gout attack. Initiation of this medication during an acute flare is not typically recommended, as serum uric acid fluctuations may intensify the inflammation.

Blueprint Task: Pharmaceutical Therapeutics

Cognitive Level: Apply

70. Cauda equina syndrome

Blueprint Task: History Taking and Performing Physical Examination

Cognitive Level: Recall

71. Triplane

A triplane fracture has a unique fracture distribution, only occurring during physeal closure affecting mainly adolescent patients. Radiographs will reveal an SH II fracture pattern on lateral views and an SH III pattern on AP views.

Blueprint Task: Formulating Most Likely Diagnosis

Cognitive Level: Apply

72. Bracing

Thoracolumbar-sacral orthosis (TLSO) is recommended at a Cobb angle starting at 25° in skeletally immature patients.

Blueprint Task: Clinical Intervention

Cognitive Level: Apply

73. A patient presents with pain and swelling of the upper extremity associated with venous thoracic outlet syndrome. What other primary physical exam finding would be expected on the affected side?

74. What prophylactic antibiotic is preferred following an open fracture without gross contamination?

75. Compression of which nerve root results in weakness with plantar flexion at the ankle and loss of the Achilles reflex?

76. A 13-year-old boy presents to the clinic with left groin pain radiating to the thigh, worsening over the last month. He denies injury but is now unable to weigh-bear on the left lower extremity. The patient has an increased BMI and is afebrile. Examination of the left lower extremity is without erythema, swelling, or warmth. Range of motion is diminished in the left hip with attempts to abduct, flex, and internally rotate. The epiphysis no longer aligns with the metaphysis on plain radiographs. What is the primary treatment recommendation?

(*See answers next page.*)

73. Discoloration

Thoracic outlet syndrome is compression of the brachial plexus or subclavian vessels between the first rib and the shoulder girdle, which worsens with overhead motion. Venous thoracic outlet syndrome is specific to compression of the subclavian vein.

Blueprint Task: History Taking and Performing Physical Examination
Cognitive Level: Apply

74. Cephalosporin

Blueprint Task: Pharmaceutical Therapeutics
Cognitive Level: Recall

75. S1

Blueprint Task: History Taking and Performing Physical Examination
Cognitive Level: Recall

76. Emergent orthopaedic surgical referral

The clinical vignette supports the diagnosis of slipped capital femoral epiphysis (SCFE) which is a surgical emergency to prevent further slippage of the femoral head. Once a SCFE is suspected, the patient should be non-weightbearing and admitted to the hospital for surgical intervention.

Blueprint Task: Clinical Intervention
Cognitive Level: Analyze

Neurologic System

1. What term describes the impaired ability to perform rapid alternating movements indicating possible cerebellar disease?

2. A patient presents acutely following multiple traumatic stab injuries to the right side of his mid-back and spine. Physical exam reveals loss of temperature and pain sensation on the left side of his body several vertebral levels below the injury. What is the presumptive diagnosis?

3. A 55-year-old man has been experiencing episodes of severe unilateral periorbital pain with ipsilateral nasal congestion, rhinorrhea, and lacrimation lasting 20–45 minutes. Aside from sumatriptan, what other intervention will assist in aborting these attacks?

4. What medication is recommended initially to reduce recovery time during an acute multiple sclerosis exacerbation though is not effective in preventing relapses?

5. A 52-year-old man presents to the clinic with new-onset, progressive headaches, confusion, and focal weakness. What is the preferred imaging study to evaluate the potential for a brain neoplasm?

6. A 28-year-old pregnant woman presents to the clinic with an abrupt onset of left-sided facial drooping and inability to fully close her left eye. She has mild left ear pain but no rash, fever, headache, confusion, or additional weakness. Drinking and eating have been difficult. What patient education can be provided to avoid ocular injury while sleeping?

7. Rest tremor, rigidity, bradykinesia, and postural instability are cardinal motor features for what condition?

8. A 35-year-old woman with a history of breast cancer, treated with chemotherapy and radiation, presents to the emergency department with a headache and recent seizure activity. Mental status changes and focal neurologic deficits are present. She was treated with antibiotics for otitis media 3 weeks ago, though she stopped the medication early due to symptom improvement. On T2-weighted MRI, there is a hyperintense central area enclosed by a well-defined capsule with surrounding edema. What is the presumptive diagnosis?

9. What is the definitive treatment for a patient with reasonable life expectancy who has experienced intracranial bleeding secondary to an arteriovenous malformation?

1. Dysdiadochokinesia
Blueprint Task: History Taking and Performing Physical Examination
Cognitive Level: Recall

2. Incomplete spinal cord injury
The loss of temperature and pain sensation supports an injury of the spinothalamic tract.
Blueprint Task: Formulating Most Likely Diagnosis
Cognitive Level: Apply

3. High-flow oxygen
The clinical vignette supports the diagnosis of cluster headaches. High-flow oxygen delivered via a face mask is standard treatment for acute attacks.
Blueprint Task: Clinical Intervention
Cognitive Level: Analyze

4. Methylprednisolone
Blueprint Task: Pharmaceutical Therapeutics
Cognitive Level: Recall

5. MRI of brain
MRI with contrast provides detail regarding the location, size, and shape of space-occupying brain lesions and assesses for cerebral edema.
Blueprint Task: Using Diagnostic and Laboratory Studies
Cognitive Level: Apply

6. Ocular lubricating ointment and eye patch
The clinical vignette supports the diagnosis of Bell's palsy. This condition is more common during pregnancy and in patients with diabetes mellitus.
Blueprint Task: Health Maintenance, Patient Education, and Preventive Measures
Cognitive Level: Analyze

7. Parkinson's disease (PD)
Blueprint Task: Applying Basic Scientific Concepts
Cognitive Level: Recall

8. Bacterial brain abscess
Bacterial brain abscesses most commonly occur in immunocompromised individuals and are a result of contiguous spread from sinus, oropharynx, or middle ear infection.
Blueprint Task: Formulating Most Likely Diagnosis
Cognitive Level: Analyze

9. Surgery
Surgical treatment is preferred in patients with prior bleeding, increased intracranial pressure, and/or neurologic deficits.
Blueprint Task: Clinical Intervention
Cognitive Level: Apply

10. What is the name of the commonly seen immunoglobulins present on cerebrospinal fluid (CSF) analysis in patients with multiple sclerosis (MS)?

11. The clinician firmly strokes the bottom of the foot from the heel, along the lateral foot, and then toward the base of the toes. In the reflex described, what represents an abnormal response?

12. A patient presents with a history and physical exam consistent with increased intracranial pressure (ICP). The head of the bed is elevated for therapeutic benefit. What medication is recommended to decrease intravascular volume and pull water from the brain parenchyma to subsequently lower ICP?

13. The American Academy of Pediatrics (AAP) recommends autism-specific screening for all patients. A common tool used is the M-CHAT (Modified Checklist for Autism in Toddlers). For low-risk children, at what ages is it recommended by the AAP to administer this screening tool?

14. A 72-year-old man presents with his wife to the clinic with progressive cognitive impairment. He also reports episodic visual hallucinations, resting tremor, frequent falls, and fears about home invasion. His wife notes that he is excessively sleepy during the day. What is the presumptive diagnosis?

15. What ocular physical exam findings are associated with cluster headaches?

16. An immunocompetent patient with osteoarthritis and hypercholesterolemia is being evaluated for presumed meningitis. Current medications include a daily multivitamin, ibuprofen, fish oil, and atorvastatin. Cerebrospinal fluid (CSF) analysis reveals normal glucose, protein, and cell count. The CSF WBC is <300 and culture and gram stain are negative. What is the next most appropriate step in the management of the presumptive diagnosis?

17. A 23-year-old woman presents to the clinic with unilateral visual disturbance, ocular pain, and paresthesia to the lower extremities. She has had mild similar symptoms in the past that worsen with heat exposure. What is the initial imaging study to further evaluate for the presumptive diagnosis?

(*See answers next page.*)

10. Oligoclonal bands

Oligoclonal bands are immunoglobulins that represent CSF inflammation but are not specific to MS. Other classic CSF findings in MS include normal appearance, pressure, and WBC count.

Blueprint Task: *Using Diagnostic and Laboratory Studies*
Cognitive Level: *Analyze*

11. Big toe extends upward/fanning of toes

The clinical vignette defines the Babinski test. Abnormal response may be associated with CNS dysfunction but is also a primitive reflex in infants.

Blueprint Task: *History Taking and Performing Physical Examination*
Cognitive Level: *Apply*

12. Mannitol

Blueprint Task: *Pharmaceutical Therapeutics*
Cognitive Level: *Recall*

13. 18 and 24 months of age

AAP recommends routine screening (surveillance) at all preventative care visits. However, ASD-specific screening is at 18 and 24 months because ASD features are typically identifiable by this time.

Blueprint Task: *Health Maintenance, Patient Education, and Preventative Measures*
Cognitive Level: *Apply*

14. Dementia with Lewy body (DLB)

In DLB, cognitive impairment typically occurs before parkinsonism symptoms (rest tremor, rigidity, postural instability, and bradykinesia). Visual hallucinations, delusions, and difficulty sleeping are commonly seen in DLB.

Blueprint Task: *Formulating Most Likely Diagnosis*
Cognitive Level: *Apply*

15. Conjunctival injection and/or lacrimation

Blueprint Task: *History Taking and Performing Physical Examination*
Cognitive Level: *Recall*

16. Discontinue ibuprofen

The clinical vignette supports the diagnosis of aseptic meningitis. Sulfonamides, nonsteroidal anti-inflammatories, along with some monoclonal antibody therapies, may be associated with the development of aseptic meningitis.

Blueprint Task: *Clinical Intervention*
Cognitive Level: *Analyze*

17. MRI of brain

The clinical vignette supports the diagnosis of multiple sclerosis. MRI with and without contrast of brain and/or spinal cord is recommended to evaluate for plaques and other characteristic findings (McDonald criteria).

Blueprint Task: *Using Diagnostic and Laboratory Studies*
Cognitive Level: *Apply*

18. A 32-year-old woman with a history of hypothyroidism develops muscle fatigability and weakness. She is diagnosed with generalized myasthenia gravis. What is the pathophysiology of this condition?

19. A 19-year-old woman presents to the clinic with a one-day history of left-sided visual disturbance and left eye pain that worsens with extraocular movement. Clinical exam reveals a relative afferent pupillary defect. What is this classic finding?

20. A 49-year-old seamstress presents to the clinic with shaky hands while trying to perform tasks at work and home. She denies shaking at rest. Symptoms improve with small amounts of alcohol and worsen with stress. Positive paternal family history of similar symptoms. What is the typical first-line medication for the presumptive diagnosis?

21. A 4-year-old boy presents to the pediatrician for a well-child visit. His parents are concerned for intellectual delay and autistic characteristics. Historical findings include delayed speech and a motor delay with his first steps at 20 months. Physical exam reveals a long narrow face with large ears, mild hypotonia, and joint laxity. What inherited genetic syndrome should be evaluated?

22. To prevent or delay neurally mediated syncope, what measure, other than avoidance of provocative stimuli, can be employed?

23. A patient suffered a penetrating head injury with subsequent cerebral abscess. What procedure is therapeutic and will confirm the suspected pathogens?

24. What is the recommended intervention for persistent dizziness following a mild concussion, thought to result from injury to the vestibular system?

25. A 29-year-old woman with a family history of headaches presents to the clinic with episodic unilateral throbbing headaches lasting 4–24 hours that worsen with lack of sleep and chocolate. The headaches are accompanied by photophobia, phonophobia, nausea, and vomiting. Acetaminophen and NSAIDs have not been beneficial. What class of medication is recommended for the acute treatment of the presumptive diagnosis?

26. What cranial nerve is involved in Bell's palsy?

(See answers next page.)

18. Autoimmune attack to the acetylcholine receptors at the neuromuscular junction

Blueprint Task: Applying Basic Scientific Concepts
Cognitive Level: Recall

19. Marcus Gunn pupil

The clinical vignette supports the diagnosis of optic neuritis. The exam performed is a swinging flashlight test.
Blueprint Task: History Taking and Performing Physical Examination
Cognitive Level: Apply

20. Propranolol

The clinical vignette supports the diagnosis of essential tremor.
Blueprint Task: Pharmaceutical Therapeutics
Cognitive Level: Analyze

21. Fragile X

Fragile X syndrome (FXS) is the most common cause of intellectual disability in males. The clinical vignette describes the common physical exam findings and autism spectrum disorder behaviors.
Blueprint Task: Formulating Most Likely Diagnosis
Cognitive Level: Analyze

22. Isometric counterpressure maneuvers of the limbs

Isometric counterpressure maneuvers may increase central blood volume resulting in an increase in blood pressure.
Blueprint Task: Health Maintenance, Patient Education, and Preventive Measures
Cognitive Level: Apply

23. CT-guided abscess aspiration

Gram stain and culture of abscess contents allow for alteration of empiric antibiotics and aids in abscess resolution.
Blueprint Task: Using Diagnostic and Laboratory Studies
Cognitive Level: Apply

24. Targeted exercises for vestibular rehabilitation

Blueprint Task: Clinical Intervention
Cognitive Level: Recall

25. Triptans

The clinical vignette supports the diagnosis of a migraine headache. Triptans inhibit the release of vasoactive neuropeptides. Trigger avoidance is also recommended.
Blueprint Task: Pharmaceutical Therapeutics
Cognitive Level: Analyze

26. Cranial nerve VII (facial nerve)

Blueprint Task: History Taking and Performing Physical Examination
Cognitive Level: Recall

27. An 8-year-old with Down syndrome presents to the pediatrician for a sports physical to participate in the Special Olympics. Screening for what spinal condition must be completed prior to clearance for contact sports?

28. A pitcher was struck on the side of the head by a foul ball and lost consciousness for several minutes. When he awoke, he knew his name and could recall the date and his current location. By the time he arrived at the emergency department, he was disoriented and not moving his right side. Which vascular structure was most likely injured?

29. A 43-year-old woman presents with intermittent pain in her elbow and paresthesia over the medial aspect of her hand, along with half of the fourth and entire fifth finger. Physical exam reveals a positive Tinel's test at the elbow and atrophy of the hypothenar muscle. What diagnostic study would demonstrate the severity of the presumptive diagnosis?

30. A mother and father present with their 2-week-old newborn for a well-child exam, asking when their baby will begin smiling responsively. At what age is this developmental milestone expected?

31. A 38-year-old woman experiences paresthesia and electrical shock sensations down her back, arms, and legs when asked to flex the neck. What is the sign associated with this abnormal physical exam finding?

32. A 4-week-old infant is transferred by EMS to the emergency department with an acute seizure. The baby is afebrile with no known health problems at birth. A CT scan of the head demonstrates an acute subdural hematoma. What other imaging should be ordered?

33. A patient arrives at the emergency department in status epilepticus. He is intubated with intravenous line placement. He has received 50% dextrose, 50 mL intravenously (IV) while en route. What is the most appropriate medication to administer at this point in his care?

(*See answers next page.*)

27. Atlantoaxial instability (AAI)

AAI is more common in patients with Down syndrome. American Academy of Pediatrics (AAP) Committee on Genetics and the AAP Committee on Sports Medicine and Fitness recommends neurological assessment and screening for atlantoaxial instability, subluxation, or dislocation. Special Olympics provides screening requirements for patients with Down Syndrome for AAI and guidelines for participation in sports with higher risk of cervical spinal trauma.

Blueprint Task: Applying Basic Scientific Concepts
Cognitive Level: Apply

28. Middle meningeal artery

The clinical vignette supports the diagnosis of an epidural hematoma, which is commonly caused by injury or tearing of the middle meningeal artery. It can manifest as a lucid interval followed by rapid neurologic deterioration.

Blueprint Task: Formulating Most Likely Diagnosis
Cognitive Level: Analyze

29. Electrodiagnostic nerve conduction study

The clinical vignette supports the diagnosis of cubital tunnel syndrome.

Blueprint Task: Using Diagnostic and Laboratory Studies
Cognitive Level: Analyze

30. By 2 months of age

Blueprint Task: Health Maintenance, Patient Education, and Preventive Measures
Cognitive Level: Recall

31. Lhermitte sign

A positive Lhermitte sign represents spinal cord dysfunction and can be seen in multiple sclerosis, cervical radiculopathy, and other conditions.

Blueprint Task: History Taking and Performing Physical Examination
Cognitive Level: Apply

32. Skeletal survey radiographs

The clinical vignette supports the diagnosis of non-accidental head trauma. Additional studies, such as radiography, complete blood count, complete metabolic panel, and coagulation studies, are necessary to evaluate for bony injuries and to screen for abdominal trauma and bleeding disorders.

Blueprint Task: Clinical Intervention
Cognitive Level: Apply

33. Lorazepam

The goal is to halt seizure activity. A bolus of lorazepam is recommended and repeated once in 10 minutes if needed. If intravenous access is not established, midazolam may be given intramuscularly or diazepam rectally.

Blueprint Task: Pharmaceutical Therapeutics
Cognitive Level: Apply

34. At what age range is the peak incidence of death of an infant prior to one year of age from an unknown cause?

35. What term is defined by involuntary, automatic behaviors, such as "picking" hand movements or lip-smacking that classically occur in focal seizures with impaired awareness?

36. A healthy 10-year-old boy presents to the clinic because his parents are concerned with increasing frequency of repetitive movements such as shoulder shrugging and blinking over the last few years. Additionally, he frequently clears his throat and grunts. There has been no concerns with the boy's academic performance and socialization; however, teachers mention difficulty focusing and inattentiveness. What is the presumptive diagnosis?

37. In a patient with decompression sickness and neurologic changes from a suspected arterial embolism, besides tissue profusion with IV fluids, what additional therapy is recommended?

38. A 57-year-old man presents to the emergency department with a headache that began 8 hours earlier while hiking and is described as "the worst headache of my life." He denies recent trauma and reports nausea and neck stiffness. CT scan of the head without contrast is negative for hemorrhage. What is the next most appropriate diagnostic study to obtain to support the presumptive diagnosis?

39. In a patient diagnosed with atrial fibrillation, what scoring system is widely used to determine the need for chronic anticoagulation to decrease stroke risk?

40. A 53-year-old woman presents to the clinic with worsening numbness and tingling in several of her fingers in both hands. On physical exam, her symptoms are exacerbated by pressing the dorsum of both hands together while maintaining full wrist flexion. Which nerve is compressed during this specialized test?

41. In an adult patient with suspected pneumococcal meningitis, what medication should be given along with, or 15–20 minutes prior to, empiric antibiotics?

(See answers next page.)

34. 2–4 months
The clinical vignette supports the diagnosis of sudden infant death syndrome (SIDS). Preventative strategies include maternal tobacco avoidance, placing the infant on their back to sleep in a crib with no pillows or toys, room sharing, breastfeeding, and avoiding infant second-hand smoke exposure.
Blueprint Task: Health Maintenance, Patient Education, and Preventive Measures
Cognitive Level: Analyze

35. Automatisms
Blueprint Task: Applying Basic Scientific Concepts
Cognitive Level: Recall

36. Tourette syndrome (TS)
TS commonly presents in childhood and includes a combination of motor and vocal tics. Comorbid conditions such as attention deficit hyperactivity disorder (ADHD), obsessive-compulsive disorder (OCD), learning disabilities, and other behavioral concerns may be present.
Blueprint Task: Formulating Most Likely Diagnosis
Cognitive Level: Apply

37. Hyperbaric oxygen
Hyperbaric oxygen is utilized for recompression and to avoid relapse of symptoms.
Blueprint Task: Clinical Intervention
Cognitive Level: Apply

38. Lumbar puncture
The clinical vignette supports the diagnosis of subarachnoid hemorrhage. The acute presentation of a severe headache coupled with neck stiffness warrants a CT scan, which, if negative, should be followed by lumbar puncture looking for xanthochromia or blood in the cerebrospinal fluid.
Blueprint Task: Using Diagnostic and Laboratory Studies
Cognitive Level: Analyze

39. CHA_2DS_2-VASc score
Blueprint Task: Health Maintenance, Patient Education, and Preventive Measures
Cognitive Level: Recall

40. Median
The clinical vignette supports the diagnosis of carpal tunnel syndrome. Phalen's test assesses median nerve compression.
Blueprint Task: History Taking and Performing Physical Examination
Cognitive Level: Analyze

41. IV dexamethasone
Dexamethasone has been shown to decrease morbidity and mortality in patients with pneumococcal meningitis.
Blueprint Task: Pharmaceutical Therapeutics
Cognitive Level: Apply

42. What cranial nerves (CN) are evaluated during an assessment of extraocular movements (EOMs)?

43. A 35-year-old man who sustained a sprain injury to his left wrist and hand 3 weeks ago presents with worsening "burning" pain exacerbated with a light touch. Physical exam reveals localized sweating over the left wrist and hand while at rest and coolness of the area when compared to the right hand. Thenar and hypothenar atrophy are noted. What is the most likely diagnosis?

44. A 24-year-old man with no prior history of seizure presents to the emergency department following a witnessed seizure. The patient exhibits no signs of infection or other related symptoms. MRI of the brain shows no lesions, and his complete blood count, complete metabolic panel, and liver tests are within normal limits. What study should be considered next in the management of this condition?

45. What vitamin is necessary during pregnancy to decrease the risk of neural tube defects?

46. An 18-month-old is brought to the clinic by his mother to establish as a new patient. He missed his 12 and 15-month well-child visits at a previous clinic. The mother reports that her child has not verbalized a single word since birth. Along with thorough history, physical, and immunization update, what other intervention is the most appropriate course of action?

47. A patient with severe spasticity secondary to cerebral palsy is being treated with an implanted intrathecal pump (ITP) containing baclofen. He presents to the emergency department with increased motor tone, pruritis, and malignant hyperthermia. What is the presumptive diagnosis?

48. The clinician asks the patient to close their eyes while drawing a number on the palm with a reflex hammer. What is the purpose of this specialized physical exam test?

49. What area of the brain is most likely affected in a patient with symptoms of a stroke that include extreme vertigo, nausea, vomiting, and neck pain?

(See answers next page.)

42. III, IV, VI
Blueprint Task: Applying Basic Scientific Concepts
Cognitive Level: Recall

43. Complex regional pain syndrome (CRPS)
CRPS occurs following a tissue injury and can result in painful and distressing sensory, vasomotor, motor (trophic), and sudomotor signs and symptoms in the affected limb.
Blueprint Task: Formulating Most Likely Diagnosis
Cognitive Level: Apply

44. Electroencephalography (EEG)
Following a solitary seizure, EEG can identify abnormalities that aid in the determination of risk of seizure recurrence.
Blueprint Task: Using Diagnostic and Laboratory Studies
Cognitive Level: Apply

45. Folic acid
Blueprint Task: Clinical Intervention
Cognitive Level: Recall

46. Referral for neurodevelopmental evaluation
The speech delay warrants further evaluation. A neurodevelopmental evaluation commonly involves a multidisciplinary team that may include clinicians, psychologists, occupational therapists, speech language pathologists, and education specialists. Close follow-up is recommended.
Blueprint Task: Health Maintenance, Patient Education, and Preventive Measures
Cognitive Level: Apply

47. Baclofen withdrawal
Baclofen withdrawal can occur in patients with ITPs containing baclofen due to pump malfunction or dislodgement of the catheter. This is a life-threatening condition that may present with hypotension, seizures, pruritis, increased motor tone, and malignant hyperthermia.
Blueprint Task: Pharmaceutical Therapeutics
Cognitive Level: Apply

48. Assess for discriminative sensation
The specialized test described in the clinical vignette is graphesthesia.
Blueprint Task: History Taking and Performing Physical Examination
Cognitive Level: Apply

49. Cerebellum
Cerebellar infarct is especially important to detect early due to risk of acute rise in intra-cranial pressure and subsequent brain stem compression.
Blueprint Task: Formulating Most Likely Diagnosis
Cognitive Level: Apply

50. A 32-year-old woman who recently had an increase in her selective serotonin reuptake inhibitor (SSRI) presents to the emergency department with agitation, hyperreflexia, akathisia, elevated blood pressure, temperature, and pulse. The medication list also includes tramadol and sumatriptan. What are the most sensitive criteria used to evaluate for the presumptive diagnosis?

51. A patient presents to the clinic with low back pain that radiates down the left lower extremity in an L4-L5 dermatomal pattern. What imaging study would best exhibit disc herniation and/or spinal nerve compression?

52. A 19-year-old college student presents with a 2-day history of worsening fever, headache, photophobia, and nuchal rigidity. The clinician flexes the patient's neck, which causes pain and flexion of his hips and knees. What is this physical exam test?

53. A 44-year-old woman is intubated in the intensive care unit due to neuromuscular respiratory failure secondary to Guillain-Barré syndrome. What pharmacologic intervention is recommended?

54. What is the most common primary intracranial tumor?

55. What type of paralysis would be expected in patients with encephalitis due to West Nile virus?

56. A 35-year-old man presents with progressive dementia along with chorea. CT of the brain shows cerebral atrophy. The patient reports that his father had similar symptoms and died at a young age, though he is not sure of his diagnosis. Genetic testing shows an abnormality on chromosome 4. What is the presumptive diagnosis?

57. What is the primary and emergent clinical intervention that should be performed on a patient with a severe injury and Glasgow coma score of <8?

58. A 6-year-old boy is seen by his pediatrician after his parents and teacher note recurrent episodes of brief lapses in attention whereby the boy gazes off into the distance for several seconds while blinking rapidly and unresponsive to the environment. After these occurrences, he is alert and awake. What is the presumptive diagnosis?

(See answers next page.)

50. Hunter serotonin toxicity criteria

The clinical vignette supports the diagnosis of serotonin syndrome.

Blueprint Task: Applying Basic Scientific Concepts
Cognitive Level: Analyze

51. MRI of lumbar spine

Blueprint Task: Using Diagnostic and Laboratory Studies
Cognitive Level: Recall

52. Brudzinski

The clinical vignette supports the diagnosis of meningitis. A positive Brudzinski sign represents meningeal irritation.

Blueprint Task: History Taking and Performing Physical Examination
Cognitive Level: *Apply*

53. Intravenous immune globulin (IVIG)

IVIG is recommended in clinically severe and rapidly progressive cases of Guillain-Barré syndrome.

Blueprint Task: Pharmaceutical Therapeutics
Cognitive Level: Apply

54. Meningioma

Blueprint Task: Applying Basic Scientific Concepts
Cognitive Level: Recall

55. Acute, asymmetric flaccid paralysis

Other physical exam findings in patients with encephalitis secondary to West Nile virus include fever, altered mental status, tremors, seizures, and cranial nerve palsies.

Blueprint Task: History Taking and Performing Physical Examination
Cognitive Level: Apply

56. Huntington's disease

Huntington's disease is an autosomal dominant genetic disorder that is potentially fatal. Progressive behavioral changes and dyskinesia are common manifestations.

Blueprint Task: Formulating Most Likely Diagnosis
Cognitive Level: Analyze

57. Intubation

Blueprint Task: Clinical Intervention
Cognitive Level: Recall

58. Absence seizures

Brief episodes that may appear to resemble daydreaming, with normal posture and no post-ictal period, are indicative of absence seizures. Further evaluation with electroencephalogram is recommended.

Blueprint Task: Formulating Most Likely Diagnosis
Cognitive Level: Apply

59. A patient with type 2 diabetes has sensitivity to touch and burning pain in his feet that is worse at night. The distribution of pain is in a stocking-glove pattern that extends to the bilateral calves. A trial of nortriptyline provides minimal relief. What class of adjunct medication is indicated to improve pain?

60. What clinical and first-line pharmacologic interventions should be considered to improve function and quality of life in a patient newly diagnosed with Alzheimer's disease?

61. A patient sustained a severe thoracic spinal cord injury (SCI) 3 hours ago. The patient is hypotensive, bradycardic, and hypothermic. What other two physical exam findings, below the level of the injury, would support the diagnosis of spinal shock?

62. Four months after suffering a mild traumatic brain injury, a 27-year-old woman reports symptoms of headaches, dizziness, irritability, insomnia, and problems with memory. What is the most likely presumptive diagnosis?

63. A 55-year-old man with a history of daily heavy alcohol use for the past 2 years abruptly discontinued drinking after losing his job. He presents with confusion, agitation, and visual hallucinations. Metabolic and electrolyte abnormalities are corrected. What class of medication should be considered to help prevent the progression of the presumptive diagnosis?

64. What is the greatest risk factor for dementia?

65. A 35-year-old man presents with recurrent headaches for several months that are described as band-like and tight on both sides of his head. He denies fever, nausea, vomiting, photophobia, aura, phonophobia, or throbbing. Movement does not exacerbate symptoms. What type of headache is he most likely experiencing?

66. The Mini-Mental State Exam (MMSE) is a brief, 30-point in-office neurologic screening tool for patients presenting with cognitive impairment. This is commonly used to evaluate orientation, registration, recall, and what other fundamental component?

(See answers next page.)

59. Anti-convulsant

The clinical vignette supports the diagnosis of diabetic peripheral neuropathy. Following a trial of tricyclic anti-depressants, anti-convulsants such as gabapentin or pregabalin as adjunct or sole therapy can often reduce neuropathic pain.

Blueprint Task: *Pharmaceutical Therapeutics*
Cognitive Level: *Apply*

60. Memory aides and cholinesterase inhibitors

Blueprint Task: *Clinical Intervention*
Cognitive Level: *Recall*

61. Decreased muscle tone and areflexia

Patients with a severe SCI may initially present with hypertension followed by the above findings.

Blueprint Task: *History Taking and Performing Physical Examination*
Cognitive Level: *Apply*

62. Postconcussion syndrome

Postconcussion syndrome involves a combination of cognitive, emotional, and physical symptoms following traumatic brain injury. Neuropsychological testing is critical in diagnosis and treatment.

Blueprint Task: *Formulating Most Likely Diagnosis*
Cognitive Level: *Apply*

63. Benzodiazepine

The clinical vignette supports the diagnosis of delirium tremens. Benzodiazepines are effective in preventing progression.

Blueprint Task: *Pharmaceutical Therapeutics*
Cognitive Level: *Apply*

64. Advancing age

Blueprint Task: *History Taking and Performing Physical Examination*
Cognitive Level: *Recall*

65. Tension

In differentiating tension-type headaches from migraine headaches, the above key features can aid in clinical diagnosis. Other considerations include family history and triggers such as bright lights, sounds, and hormonal fluctuations.

Blueprint Task: *Formulating Most Likely Diagnosis*
Cognitive Level: *Apply*

66. Language

Blueprint Task: *Clinical Intervention*
Cognitive Level: *Recall*

Psychiatry/Behavioral Science

1. What is the mood state that includes hyperactivity, irritability, flight of ideas, distractibility, and decreased need for sleep that does not cause significant functional impairment?

2. A 34-year-old man with a BMI of 30 kg/m² and a family history of type 2 diabetes and hyperlipidemia is started on an antipsychotic agent. What laboratory testing is recommended due to the potential metabolic effects of this medication class?

3. A 25-year-old man was recently started on haloperidol. He presents to the emergency department with lead pipe rigidity, elevated temperature, confusion, irritability, sweating, and rapid pulse. What is the most likely diagnosis?

4. A combat veteran presents to the clinic with many months of increasing, recurrent nightmares and flashbacks related to the traumatic events of his military experiences from over a year ago. He feels down, anxious, isolated, and is struggling to function at work. He reports that he has not had a restful sleep in months. What is the recommended non pharmacological therapy for the presumptive diagnosis?

5. A previously healthy 19-year-old man presents to the emergency department with social detachment along with delusions and hallucinations over the last 8 months. His mother reports that he got terminated from his job, has difficulty concentrating, and does not have interest in things he used to enjoy. The drug screen is negative, and the patient reports no history of illicit drug use. What is the first-line class of medication for acute and chronic symptoms associated with the presumptive diagnosis?

6. What is the most prevalent form of maltreatment in the elderly population defined by a caregiver's failure to provide basic needs such as withholding food, clothing, or medical care?

7. A 12-year-old boy is brought to the clinic by his mother, who reports years of difficulty maintaining focused attention, restlessness, and impulsivity since early elementary school. During the past few years, these symptoms started interfering with home life, school, and sports. What class of medication is most effective for the presumptive diagnosis?

1. Hypomanic episode

Blueprint Task: History Taking and Performing Physical Examination
Cognitive Level: Recall

2. Fasting blood sugar and lipid panel

For patients on an antipsychotic agent, it is recommended to closely monitor weight and encourage diet and exercise because this class of drug can cause weight gain. The clinician must monitor for signs of insulin resistance and hyperlipidemia, which are side effects of the drug. Fasting blood sugar and lipid evaluation are recommended at 3- to 6-month intervals.

Blueprint Task: Using Diagnostic and Laboratory Studies
Cognitive Level: Apply

3. Neuroleptic malignant syndrome (NMS)

NMS is represented by the tetrad of mental status change, muscle rigidity, fever, and autonomic instability. All antipsychotic medications have the potential to cause NMS; however, typical antipsychotics such as haloperidol have a greater risk.

Blueprint Task: Formulating Most Likely Diagnosis
Cognitive Level: Analyze

4. Trauma-focused psychotherapy

The clinical vignette supports the diagnosis of post-traumatic stress disorder (PTSD). Examples of techniques used in trauma-focused psychotherapy include relaxation, visualization, and cognitive reframing.

Blueprint Task: Clinical Intervention
Cognitive Level: Analyze

5. Antipsychotics

The clinical vignette supports the diagnosis of schizophrenia.
Blueprint Task: Pharmaceutical Therapeutics
Cognitive Level: Analyze

6. Elder neglect

Blueprint Task: Applying Basic Scientific Concepts
Cognitive Level: Recall

7. Stimulants

The clinical vignette supports the diagnosis of attention deficit hyperactivity disorder (ADHD).

Blueprint Task: Pharmaceutical Therapeutics
Cognitive Level: Apply

8. A mother brings her 9-year-old son into the clinic for evaluation. She reports that her son is rebellious and disobedient. Teachers and family members report concerns that the child has been irritable, argumentative, and frequently loses his temper. His actions do not break the law, but his behavior is impacting home life and the ability to learn at school. What is the most likely diagnosis?

9. A 3-year-old boy is undergoing extensive evaluation for autism spectrum disorder (ASD). His home was built over 50 years ago, and the mother reports constant home renovation projects. She also has a hobby of making glazed pottery in the home. Based on these home environment risk factors, what laboratory test should be considered during the evaluation for ASD?

10. What type of personality disorder is best described during the history as extensive strained relationships, lack of empathy, focus on power, excessive desire for admiration, and grandiosity?

11. The mother of a 13-year-old boy with conduct disorder asks, "Is there a medication that can take away my son's disruptive and aggressive behavior?" What patient education should be provided regarding pharmacological therapy for this condition?

12. While not a component of the diagnostic criteria for anorexia nervosa, what menstrual irregularity is a common finding in females of child-bearing age with this condition?

13. A 39-year-old woman left her abusive husband one year ago. She presents to the clinic reporting that even though she feels safe, she continues to relive the distressing events with recurring, persistent emotionally painful dreams and flashbacks. She no longer feels close with friends and has felt down and anxious. She voices uncertainty about even considering future relationships. What is the presumptive diagnosis?

14. A 36-year-old healthy man presents to the clinic with depressive symptoms, malaise, and fatigue. In addition to thyroid function tests, what other laboratory test is recommended in the evaluation of this patient?

(See answers next page.)

8. Oppositional defiant disorder (ODD)

ODD, unlike conduct disorder (CD), does not typically include severe aggression, destruction, or unlawful behavior; however, the characteristics described in the clinical vignette are recurrent and persistent.

Blueprint Task: Formulating Most Likely Diagnosis
Cognitive Level: Apply

9. Lead level

Lead toxicity may lead to cognitive impairment, language delay, behavior problems, and additional issues. Consideration of lead toxicity in the evaluation of ASD is important in high-risk patients.

Blueprint Task: Using Diagnostic and Laboratory Studies
Cognitive Level: Apply

10. Narcissistic

Blueprint Task: History Taking and Performing Physical Examination
Cognitive Level: Recall

11. Motivated aggression is often refractory to pharmacological therapy

Pharmaceutical treatment may be helpful for patients with conduct disorder who also have other psychiatric conditions such as attention deficit hyperactivity disorder (ADHD) or depression. However, to best manage the aggressive behavior, psychotherapy is the first-line recommendation.

Blueprint Task: Health Maintenance, Patient Education, and Preventive Measures
Cognitive Level: Apply

12. Amenorrhea

Blueprint Task: Applying Basic Scientific Concepts
Cognitive Level: Recall

13. Posttraumatic stress disorder (PTSD)

Patients with PTSD may experience emotional detachment. Forms of abuse may vary and include, but are not limited to, sexual, mental, and physical.

Blueprint Task: Formulating Most Likely Diagnosis
Cognitive Level: Apply

14. Complete blood count (CBC)

CBC and thyroid function tests will evaluate the possibility of anemia and hypothyroidism in a patient with depressive symptoms.

Blueprint Task: Using Diagnostic and Laboratory Studies
Cognitive Level: Apply

15. A 19-year-old woman has a 2-year history of binge eating multiple times per week followed by self-induced purging to avoid weight gain. If the oral exam reveals an abnormality, what would be the most likely finding?

16. A 29-year-old woman presents with an intense fear of spiders. She recently purchased a home and is having difficulty sleeping and functioning because of her extreme fear. What is the treatment of choice for the presumptive diagnosis?

17. What medication inhibits aldehyde dehydrogenase and with alcohol consumption causes unpleasant effects such as palpitations, headache, nausea, and vomiting?

18. What population is at the highest risk for completed suicide?

19. A 45-year-old healthy man presents to the clinic reporting auditory hallucinations over the last 6 months. There is no history of drug use or previous mental illness. History and physical exam are nondefinitive. What imaging is recommended?

20. A 25-year-old woman with a history of panic disorder reports an irritational fear of being trapped or unable to escape a situation that insights a panic attack. What is the term that describes this historical finding?

21. A 31-year-old woman is diagnosed with major depressive disorder and is prescribed fluoxetine. During a follow-up visit, she describes mild nausea since starting this medication. What patient education is recommended to reduce gastrointestinal symptoms?

22. A 50-year-old man presents to the clinic with extreme somnolence that increases throughout the day and affects his ability to work and function. He also describes abrupt episodes of muscle weakness and dream-like hallucinations. What initial diagnostic study is recommended to evaluate for the suspected diagnosis?

(See answers next page.)

15. Dental erosion

The clinical vignette supports bulimia nervosa. Physical exam is often normal in patients with this condition; however, dental erosion and parotid gland enlargement may be present.

Blueprint Task: History Taking and Performing Physical Examination

Cognitive Level: Apply

16. Cognitive behavioral psychotherapy with exposure

The clinical vignette supports the diagnosis of specific phobia. Cognitive behavioral psychotherapy often includes relaxation training, visualization, and desensitization.

Blueprint Task: Clinical Intervention

Cognitive Level: Analyze

17. Disulfiram

Blueprint Task: Pharmaceutical Therapeutics

Cognitive Level: Recall

18. Elderly male

Blueprint Task: Applying Basic Scientific Concepts

Cognitive Level: Recall

19. MRI of brain

Brain MRI is beneficial to evaluate for structural abnormalities in patients with acute mental status changes or psychotic episodes. This case warrants imaging due to age at onset and no history of drug use or previous mental illness.

Blueprint Task: Using Diagnostic and Laboratory Studies

Cognitive Level: Apply

20. Agoraphobia

Blueprint Task: History Taking and Performing Physical Examination

Cognitive Level: Recall

21. Take medication with food

Fluoxetine is a selective serotonin reuptake inhibitor (SSRI); gastrointestinal side effects such as nausea and vomiting are common and may improve by taking medication with food.

Blueprint Task: Health Maintenance, Patient Education, and Preventive Measures

Cognitive Level: Apply

22. Polysomnogram

The clinical vignette supports the diagnosis of narcolepsy. Cataplexy, a form of narcolepsy, causes abrupt transient muscle weakness without altered consciousness and is usually precipitated by intense emotions.

Blueprint Task: Clinical Intervention

Cognitive Level: Analyze

23. What is the most commonly used illicit drug in the United States?

24. A 26-year-old woman with a family history of depression presents to the clinic report-ing repetitive, unexpected occurrences of severe fear lasting <1 hour over the last 6 months. During the episodes, she also experiences palpitations, dyspnea, shakiness, and a fear of dying. For months she has been concerned about having an attack, which has caused her to limit social exposure. What is the most likely diagnosis?

25. The clinician is evaluating a young woman for obsessive compulsive disorder. On physical exam, patchy loss of hair is present. What is the most likely cause of this physi-cal exam finding?

26. A 23-year-old woman presents to the clinic with sadness, sleep disturbance, and an increased appetite that occur seasonally during the fall and winter. She was prescribed selective serotonin reuptake inhibitors (SSRIs). What nonpharmacological therapy can be initiated daily during these seasons?

27. Personality disorders have been grouped into three clusters: A, B, and C. Which cluster includes antisocial, borderline, histrionic, and narcissistic types?

28. A patient is diagnosed with dissociative disorder. Her friend takes a neuroleptic medi-cation for a different mental health diagnosis, and the patient asks if this medication would be an option also for her condition. What patient education is recommended when considering this class of medication for dissociative disorder?

29. A 72-year-old man with a history of major depressive disorder presents to the emer-gency department reporting that he feels hopeless and helpless. He states that he wants to end his life and verbalizes the way in which he plans to commit suicide. What is the disposition plan for this patient?

30. A 27-year-old woman with a BMI of 33 kg/m^2 describes uncontrollable episodes of rapidly eating large amounts of food in one sitting. These episodes occur 3 to 4 times per week for the last 6 months. She denies increased hunger and reports feeling uncom-fortably full after each event. She displays feelings of guilt and embarrassment. What historical feature classically differentiates the presumptive diagnosis from bulimia nervosa?

(See answers next page.)

23. Marijuana
Blueprint Task: Applying Basic Scientific Concepts
Cognitive Level: Recall

24. Panic disorder
Panic attacks typically are unpredictable and have a rapid onset. Panic disorders are commonly associated with other psychiatric conditions, such as major depression.
Blueprint Task: Formulating Most Likely Diagnosis
Cognitive Level: Apply

25. Trichotillomania
Trichotillomania is a persistent urge to repetitively pull out hair and is more common in the female population.
Blueprint Task: History Taking and Performing Physical Examination
Cognitive Level: Apply

26. Light therapy
The clinical vignette supports the diagnosis of seasonal affective disorder (SAD). Light therapy may trigger mania symptoms, so screening for bipolar disorder is important.
Blueprint Task: Clinical Intervention
Cognitive Level: Apply

27. Cluster B
Blueprint Task: Applying Basic Scientific Concepts
Cognitive Level: Recall

28. Neuroleptic medications are contraindicated
Neuroleptic medications are not an effective treatment option for patients with dissociative disorder and may exacerbate dissociative symptoms.
Blueprint Task: Health Maintenance, Patient Education, and Preventive Measures
Cognitive Level: Apply

29. Admit as an acute psychiatric emergency
The clinical vignette describes suicidal ideation with plan which should be addressed emergently.
Blueprint Task: Clinical Intervention
Cognitive Level: Apply

30. Behaviors to prevent weight gain
The clinical vignette describes binge-eating disorder, which is more common than bulimia nervosa. Binge-eating lacks compensatory behavior such as purging, laxatives, fasting, or excessive exercise following eating to prevent weight gain.
Blueprint Task: History Taking and Performing Physical Examination
Cognitive Level: Analyze

31. What patient education should initially be discussed in the management of insomnia?

32. A 30-year-old woman with a family history of depression reports chronic anhedonia and sadness for at least the last 2 to 3 years. Her symptoms have been persistent without any thoughts of harm to self or others. What is the presumptive diagnosis?

33. A jazz artist is prescribed a medication to help with "performance anxiety." She is advised to medicate 2 hours prior to the concert to ease anxiety symptoms of sweating, palpitations, and tremor. What is the most likely non-habit-forming class of medication used to treat the presumptive diagnosis?

34. A 16-year-old adolescent presents to the clinic with irritability, moodiness, and anxiety that began within weeks after his close friend unexpectedly passed away. His grades are declining in school, and he is less successful in sports but is still able to participate in both. There is no history of preexisting mental health diagnoses, substance abuse, or thoughts of harm. What is the presumptive diagnosis?

35. What is the legal limit of blood ethanol concentration for operating a motor vehicle in most states in the United States?

36. In an adolescent patient with depressed mood, what oral retinoid medication has been associated with depression and should be elicited for during the medical history?

37. What is a common neurodevelopmental disorder represented by inattention and/or hyperactivity-impulsivity?

38. What is the primary pharmacological management for an opioid overdose?

(See answers next page.)

31. Sleep hygiene
Blueprint Task: Health Maintenance, Patient Education, and Preventive Measures
Cognitive Level: Recall

32. Persistent depressive disorder
Persistent depressive disorder (also known as dysthymia) tends to have less severe symptoms than major depressive disorder, but symptoms remain for longer periods. Anhedonia is loss of interest and pleasure in activities that were previously enjoyable.
Blueprint Task: Formulating Most Likely Diagnosis
Cognitive Level: Apply

33. Beta-blockers
The clinical vignette describes the diagnosis of phobic disorder. Propranolol is a commonly used beta-blocker in patients with this diagnosis.
Blueprint Task: Pharmaceutical Therapeutics
Cognitive Level: Apply

34. Adjustment disorder
Additional common factors contributing to adjustment disorder in children include difficult family events such as divorce, illness, or trauma. Reassurance, patience, and compassion to the patient and family are recommended. Symptoms diminish within 6 months.
Blueprint Task: Formulating Most Likely Diagnosis
Cognitive Level: Apply

35. 0.08 g/dL
Blueprint Task: Using Diagnostic and Laboratory Studies
Cognitive Level: Recall

36. Isotretinoin
Isotretinoin can be prescribed for acne management. Follow-up visit for patients taking isotretinoin include monitoring for psychiatric symptoms.
Blueprint Task: History Taking and Performing Physical Examination
Cognitive Level: Apply

37. Attention deficit hyperactivity disorder (ADHD)
Blueprint Task: Applying Basic Scientific Concepts
Cognitive Level: Recall

38. Naloxone
Blueprint Task: Pharmaceutical Therapeutics
Cognitive Level: Recall

39. The parents of a 6-year-old boy report concerns of sleep issues. Their child abruptly sits up an hour or so after falling asleep and cries out. He is sweaty, breathing rapidly, and looks terrified. The parents are baffled that the child does not remember the episode in the morning. What patient education is recommended for the most likely condition?

40. What electrocardiogram abnormality may be identified in a patient with a tricyclic anti-depressant overdose?

41. A 22-year-old woman presents to the clinic with a 1- to 2-year history of difficulty concentrating and feeling tense and jittery. In the last 6 months her symptoms have worsened and occur daily. She is losing sleep due to excessively worrying about small issues. She denies chest pain, shortness of breath, or suicidal ideation. What is the presumptive diagnosis?

42. What class of antidepressant medication is used for the treatment of depressive disorders, anxiety, and chronic pain syndromes such as diabetic neuropathy or fibromyalgia?

43. A 29-year-old man was brought to the emergency department due to an apparent overdose. His roommate reports that he took a large quantity of pills that were previously prescribed for short-term treatment of anxiety. On physical exam, the patient has unsteady gait and appears to be sleepy, confused, and has difficulty performing rapid alternating movements. An overdose of which class of medication would cause this clinical presentation?

44. A 24-year-old woman presents to the clinic reporting a fear of germs and contamination for the last 5 years. She admits to checking and rechecking the stove and oven to be sure they are off and repeatedly locking the doors prior to bedtime. She also reports feeling "down" and anxious. During the last 6 months, the feelings and behaviors started impacting her daily functioning. On physical exam, her hands are dry, red, and chapped. What is the presumptive diagnosis?

45. What is a commonly used nine-question tool in the evaluation and follow-up of patients with major depression?

46. An 82-year-old woman is brought to the emergency department by her husband. He reports his wife has been confused on and off over the last 24 hours, is having trouble paying attention, and has developed hallucinations. Further history reveals she has been going to the restroom more frequently with dysuria for the past 3 days. What medication is recommended to treat the presumptive diagnosis?

(*See answers next page.*)

39. Reassurance

The clinical vignette supports the diagnosis of sleep terrors. The condition is usually self-limited and occurs in young children in the first few hours of sleep. Consistent sleep hygiene with a healthy sleep schedule may improve terrors.

Blueprint Task: Health Maintenance, Patient Education, and Preventive Measures
Cognitive Level: Analyze

40. QT prolongation

Blueprint Task: Using Diagnostic and Laboratory Studies
Cognitive Level: Recall

41. Generalized anxiety disorder (GAD)

Patients with GAD do not typically experience shortness of breath, palpitations, or chest pain, which are more commonly described in individuals with panic disorder.

Blueprint Task: Formulating Most Likely Diagnosis
Cognitive Level: Apply

42. Serotonin norepinephrine reuptake inhibitors (SNRIs)

Blueprint Task: Clinical Intervention
Cognitive Level: Recall

43. Benzodiazepine

Benzodiazepine overdose may also lead to respiratory depression when combined with other medications such as opioids.

Blueprint Task: Pharmaceutical Therapeutics
Cognitive Level: Analyze

44. Obsessive compulsive disorder (OCD)

Hand findings described in the clinical vignette are secondary to excessive washing which is common in OCD. Other psychiatric disorders, such as depression and anxiety, may be present in patients with OCD.

Blueprint Task: Formulating Most Likely Diagnosis
Cognitive Level: Apply

45. Patient Health Questionnaire (PHQ-9)

Blueprint Task: Clinical Intervention
Cognitive Level: Recall

46. Empiric antibiotics

The clinical vignette supports the diagnosis of delirium likely caused by a urinary tract infection. Delirium typically presents as an acute mental status change with altered attention and awareness. Management of delirium includes identifying and managing the underlying cause.

Blueprint Task: Pharmaceutical Therapeutics
Cognitive Level: Analyze

47. What is a strong, irrational fear of a certain object or situation such as clowns or confined spaces?

48. A 16-year-old patient presents with his parents for behavioral concerns. These include starting fistfights with classmates, cruelty to animals, shoplifting, skipping school, and losing his temper easily. He has been caught destroying property and running away from home many times. The patient's behaviors began around age 10 and have intensified. What is the minimum timeframe for at least one of these behaviors to be present to meet criteria for the presumptive diagnosis?

49. A child presents to the emergency department with possible sexual abuse. Swabs for sexually transmitted infection may be obtained from the rectum, vagina, and urethra. What other location could be considered based on the history?

50. A 25-year-old woman is diagnosed with a condition that is characterized by unpredictable mood swings. She experiences periods of grandiosity, reduced need for sleep, and agitation followed by feelings of depression. What medication is considered the mainstay treatment for the presumptive diagnosis and requires blood level monitoring?

51. What term describes the incapacity to recollect critical personal information based on life events due to a traumatic exposure?

52. A 42-year-old woman reports an irresistible urge to move her legs while trying to sleep or during periods of inactivity, such as watching a movie. This has caused significant issues with quality of sleep. What abnormal lab finding is most commonly associated with the presumptive diagnosis?

53. A 45-year-old patient who has had an extensive unremarkable diagnostic workup continues to report subjective high fevers with exaggerated concerns. What disorder is characterized by self-induced or falsely represented medical symptoms?

54. A 4-year-old boy presents to the clinic with his mother to establish as a new patient. The patient has not had consistent medical care since birth. The mother reports concerns that her son has minimal eye contact, delayed language development, and lack of interest in playing with friends or communicating with family. He demands consistency with schedules and demonstrates repetitive motor movements such as lining up toys. What is the most likely diagnosis?

55. What is the most common form of non-suicidal self-injury?

(See answers next page.)

47. Specific phobia
Blueprint Task: Formulating Most Likely Diagnosis
Cognitive Level: Recall

48. 6 months
The clinical vignette supports the diagnosis of conduct disorder.
Blueprint Task: History Taking and Performing Physical Examination
Cognitive Level: Analyze

49. Pharynx
Blueprint Task: Using Diagnostic and Laboratory Studies
Cognitive Level: Recall

50. Lithium carbonate
The clinical vignette supports the diagnosis of bipolar disorder.
Blueprint Task: Pharmaceutical Therapeutics
Cognitive Level: Analyze

51. Dissociative amnesia
Blueprint Task: Formulating Most Likely Diagnosis
Cognitive Level: Recall

52. Iron deficiency
The clinical vignette supports the diagnosis of restless leg syndrome.
Blueprint Task: Using Diagnostic and Laboratory Studies
Cognitive Level: Analyze

53. Factitious disorder imposed on self
Factitious disorder imposed on self (previously termed "Munchausen syndrome") may also present with falsely represented physical and laboratory findings.
Blueprint Task: History Taking and Performing Physical Examination
Cognitive Level: Apply

54. Autism spectrum disorder (ASD)
All low-risk patients should be screened for ASD at 18 months and again at 24-30 months, with developmental surveillance occurring at every visit. Children with a higher risk for ASD may be screened earlier or at different intervals. ASD is more common in boys.
Blueprint Task: Formulating Most Likely Diagnosis
Cognitive Level: Apply

55. Cutting
Blueprint Task: History Taking and Performing Physical Examination
Cognitive Level: Recall

56. What therapy, performed under general anesthesia, uses a brief small electric current to induce a generalized seizure and appears to be most effective in patients with severe depression?

57. A woman presents to the clinic to discuss problems with moodiness and feeling "on edge" that occur cyclically once per month. A friend told her about a behavioral health condition that is associated with hormones and the menstrual cycle. Based on the presumptive diagnosis, what portion of the menstrual cycle are patients most symptomatic?

58. A patient is being treated for opioid use disorder. What effect may be induced if buprenorphine is prescribed while the patient is still actively taking opioids?

(See answers next page.)

56. Electroconvulsive therapy (ECT)
Blueprint Task: *Clinical Intervention*
Cognitive Level: *Recall*

57. Late luteal phase
The clinical vignette supports the diagnosis of premenstrual dysphoric disorder (PMDD). Premenstrual irritability is commonly experienced in the last 2 weeks of the menstrual cycle.
Blueprint Task: *Health Maintenance, Patient Education, and Preventive Measures*
Cognitive Level: *Analyze*

58. Acute withdrawal
Buprenorphine is a partial agonist that will bind preferentially as an antagonist in the presence of an agonist (opioid), leading to symptoms of withdrawal such as anxiety, diarrhea, nausea, vomiting, diaphoresis, and rhinorrhea in an opioid-dependent patient.
Blueprint Task: *Health Maintenance, Patient Education, and Preventive Measures*
Cognitive Level: *Apply*

Pulmonary System

1. What is the compression-to-ventilation ratio for two providers administering CPR on an infant?

2. A 48-year-old man with a BMI of 34 kg/m² presents to the clinic with chronic fatigue, headaches, and a history of loud snoring. What diagnostic study is recommended to confirm the most likely diagnosis?

3. A 65-year-old man with a 40-pack year tobacco history presents with chronic cough with sputum production, dyspnea on exertion, and fatigue for the past 2 years, which was not previously evaluated due to lack of insurance. Physical exam reveals distended neck veins, digital clubbing, peripheral edema, and an S3 gallop. What is the most likely diagnosis?

4. What intervention should be implemented immediately following the diagnosis of a large hemothorax?

5. A premature newborn, delivered at 29 weeks' gestation, develops tachypnea, cyanosis, and grunting. Deficiency of what substance is the pathophysiologic cause of this patient's respiratory distress shortly after birth?

6. The pneumococcal conjugate vaccine PCV13 series is routinely administered at 2, 4, 6, and 12–15 months of age. Children ≥ 2 years old who are immune-compromised or with high-risk chronic conditions are also advised to receive what additional pneumococcal vaccine?

7. A 30-year-old woman with asthma reports increased respiratory symptoms after beginning her new job at a veterinary office. She has a known sensitivity to pet dander that has been unresponsive to OTC medications and exposure modification. She is compliant with daily inhaled corticosteroid and would like to minimize bronchodilator use. What therapy may be recommended that must be administered under medical supervision?

8. Palivizumab is a monoclonal antibody recommended for high-risk infants to prophylactically protect against what virus?

(See answers next page.)

1. 15:2
Blueprint Task: Clinical Intervention
Cognitive Level: Recall

2. Overnight polysomnography
The clinical vignette supports the diagnosis of obstructive sleep apnea (OSA). Polysomnography will typically detect apnea with hypoxemia in patients with OSA.
Blueprint Task: Using Diagnostic and Laboratory Studies
Cognitive Level: Apply

3. Cor pulmonale
The clinical vignette describes a patient with chronic obstructive pulmonary disease (COPD). COPD can lead to chronic hypoxemia, which can contribute to the development of cor pulmonale.
Blueprint Task: History Taking and Performing Physical Examination
Cognitive Level: Analyze

4. Placement of a thoracostomy tube
Blueprint Task: Clinical Intervention
Cognitive Level: Recall

5. Surfactant
The clinical vignette supports the diagnosis of respiratory distress syndrome, formerly termed hyaline membrane disease. This is the most common cause of respiratory distress in premature infants.
Blueprint Task: Formulating Most Likely Diagnosis
Cognitive Level: Analyze

6. Pneumococcal polysaccharide (PPSV23) vaccine
Blueprint Task: Health Maintenance, Patient Education, and Preventive Measures
Cognitive Level: Recall

7. Immunotherapy
Immunotherapy provides desensitization. Patients must be monitored after receiving immunotherapy due to risk of systemic reaction.
Blueprint Task: Clinical Intervention
Cognitive Level: Apply

8. Respiratory syncytial virus (RSV)
Blueprint Task: Pharmaceutical Therapeutics
Cognitive Level: Recall

9. What commonly used pharmacologic smoking cessation therapy is an atypical antidepressant and is contraindicated in patients with a seizure disorder?

10. Which two classes of medication may be prescribed as a first-line treatment of Legionnaires' disease?

11. What acid–base disorder is most commonly associated with Kussmaul respirations?

12. What medication is commonly used in bronchoprovocation testing?

13. A 62-year-old man presents to the clinic with a 4-day history of productive cough and fever. Chest radiograph reveals left lower lobe consolidation. What would be heard with bronchophony over the left lower lobe based on the presumptive diagnosis?

14. What modifiable risk factor is the leading cause of pulmonary malignancy?

15. A 32-year-old patient without a history of tobacco use is diagnosed with chronic obstructive pulmonary disease (COPD). What primary laboratory test is recommended to investigate the most common cause of hereditary COPD?

16. A 62-year-old woman with congestive heart failure (CHF) presents to the emergency department with severe shortness of breath and productive cough that produces frothy, pink sputum. She denies chest pain. Physical exam reveals crackles and wheezing. What is the interpretation of the following chest radiograph?

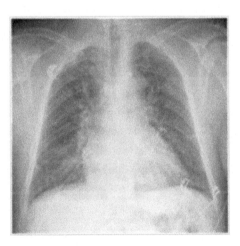

(See answers next page.)

9. Bupropion

Bupropion may lower the seizure threshold placing patients predisposed to seizures at increased risk.

Blueprint Task: Pharmaceutical Therapeutics
Cognitive Level: Apply

10. Macrolides or quinolones

Blueprint Task: Pharmaceutical Therapeutics
Cognitive Level: Recall

11. Metabolic acidosis

Kussmaul respirations are described as deep, sighing, and may be seen in conditions such as ketoacidosis.

Blueprint Task: Applying Basic Scientific Concepts
Cognitive Level: Apply

12. Methacholine

Blueprint Task: Pharmaceutical Therapeutics
Cognitive Level: Recall

13. Sounds are clear and louder

The clinical vignette supports the diagnosis of pneumonia. In a patient with consolidation and positive bronchophony, auscultation produces louder, clearer sounds in the affected area. In the absence of pulmonary abnormalities, spoken sounds are indistinct with auscultation.

Blueprint Task: History Taking and Performing Physical Examination
Cognitive Level: Analyze

14. Cigarette smoking

Blueprint Task: Applying Basic Scientific Concepts
Cognitive Level: Recall

15. Alpha-1-antitrypsin level

Alpha-1-antitrypsin deficiency, also known as antiprotease deficiency, is an inherited cause of early-onset emphysema.

Blueprint Task: Using Diagnostic and Laboratory Studies
Cognitive Level: Apply

16. Pulmonary edema

Pulmonary edema may be caused by cardiac or noncardiac conditions. The chest radiograph findings represent fluid within the interstitial and alveolar spaces.

Blueprint Task: Formulating Most Likely Diagnosis
Cognitive Level: Analyze

17. What is the most common pathogen causing bronchiolitis?

18. A healthy 33-year-old woman presents to the clinic with a 3-day history of mild cough with occasional yellow sputum. She denies fever or dyspnea. She requests antibiotics as she believes the discolored sputum is indicative of a bacterial infection. What patient education should be provided regarding the sputum?

19. What is the standard medical therapy for obstructive sleep apnea?

20. What medication is preferred in all stages of persistent asthma management?

21. What type of pneumonia is often associated with gastrointestinal manifestations and is confirmed with urinary antigen testing?

22. Sensitivity to what class of medication should be considered in a patient with chronic rhinosinusitis, nasal polyps, and asthma?

23. If CT angiogram cannot be performed, what is the next best noninvasive pulmonary imaging study for the evaluation of a pulmonary embolism?

24. A 40-year-old man presents with a cough for 8 days with recent onset of mild dyspnea and low-grade fever. The cough was initially nonproductive, but he now describes mucoid sputum. No history of asthma or previous similar illness. Physical exam reveals rhonchi that resolve with cough. Vitals are stable, and radiographs are negative. What is the most likely diagnosis?

(See answers next page.)

17. Respiratory syncytial virus (RSV)
Blueprint Task: Applying Basic Scientific Concepts
Cognitive Level: Recall

18. Discolored sputum is not indicative of bacterial infection
The clinical vignette supports the diagnosis of viral bronchitis, the most common cause of acute bronchitis. Supportive care is recommended.
Blueprint Task: Health Maintenance, Patient Education, and Preventive Measures
Cognitive Level: Apply

19. Continuous positive airway pressure (CPAP)
Blueprint Task: Clinical Intervention
Cognitive Level: Recall

20. Inhaled corticosteroids (ICS)
ICS may be used as daily monotherapy or in combination with other medications dependent on asthma severity.
Blueprint Task: Pharmaceutical Therapeutics
Cognitive Level: Apply

21. Legionella
Blueprint Task: Formulating Most Likely Diagnosis
Cognitive Level: Recall

22. Nonsteroidal anti-inflammatory drug (NSAID)
Aspirin-exacerbated respiratory disease (AERD) commonly presents as Samter triad defined by inflammation of the sinuses, nasal polyps, and asthma.
Blueprint Task: History Taking and Performing Physical Examination
Cognitive Level: Apply

23. Ventilation-perfusion (V/Q) scan
Blueprint Task: Using Diagnostic and Laboratory Studies
Cognitive Level: Recall

24. Acute bronchitis
Acute bronchitis should be considered in patients with fever, dyspnea, and cough for more than 5 days. The cough may initially be dry and later become productive. Chest radiograph helps to distinguish acute bronchitis from pneumonia.
Blueprint Task: Formulating Most Likely Diagnosis
Cognitive Level: Apply

25. What imaging study is recommended in a 63-year-old man with a 30-pack year smoking history to screen for lung cancer?

26. What therapeutic procedure is recommended for a symptomatic patient with a large malignant pleural effusion?

27. A 22-year-old woman with asthma presents to the emergency department with increasing chest tightness, progressive dyspnea, and decreased peak flow measurements. She was placed on oxygen and provided high doses of short-acting beta agonist (SABA) with minimal relief. What additional medication should be provided to this patient?

28. What is the most common bacterial pathogen causing community-acquired pneumonia (CAP) in the United States?

29. A healthy 32-year-old man began working at an aviary 6 months ago. Shortly after beginning the job, he developed cough, chills, fatigue, dyspnea, and intermittent fever. Symptoms improved during a 2-week vacation. Chest radiograph reveals features consistent with pulmonary fibrosis. If pharmacologic treatment is needed, what class of medication may accelerate the resolution of symptoms?

30. What is the characteristic sputum associated with *Klebsiella pneumoniae*?

31. A healthy 29-year-old woman presents to the clinic with chest pain that worsens with deep breaths and coughing following a viral respiratory infection. What is the most likely diagnosis?

32. What is the expected tactile fremitus finding in a patient with a large pneumothorax?

(See answers next page.)

25. Low-dose CT of chest

Blueprint Task: Health Maintenance, Patient Education, and Preventive Measures
Cognitive Level: Recall

26. Thoracentesis

Common symptoms that may necessitate treatment include dyspnea, cough, and chest pain. Asymptomatic malignant pleural effusions do not require clinical intervention.
Blueprint Task: Clinical Intervention
Cognitive Level: Apply

27. Systemic corticosteroids

The clinical vignette represents an asthma exacerbation. Corticosteroids are effective for decreasing airway obstruction, controlling asthma exacerbations, and reducing risk of relapse.
Blueprint Task: Pharmaceutical Therapeutics
Cognitive Level: Apply

28. *Streptococcus pneumoniae*

Blueprint Task: Applying Basic Scientific Concepts
Cognitive Level: Recall

29. Glucocorticoids

The clinical vignette supports the diagnosis of hypersensitivity pneumonitis, an inflammatory, immunologic reaction to the inhaled antigens from bird feces. Prior to initiating medication, environmental risk reduction is recommended.
Blueprint Task: Clinical Intervention
Cognitive Level: Analyze

30. Currant jelly

Blueprint Task: History Taking and Performing Physical Examination
Cognitive Level: Recall

31. Pleuritis

Pleuritis (also called pleurisy) is caused by irritation of the pleural lining of the lung and is often associated with viral respiratory infections.
Blueprint Task: Formulating Most Likely Diagnosis
Cognitive Level: Analyze

32. Decreased or absent tactile fremitus

Blueprint Task: History Taking and Performing Physical Examination
Cognitive Level: Recall

33. A 62-year-old man with coronary artery disease presents with orthopnea, pitting lower extremity edema, and shortness of breath. Echocardiogram reveals reduced ejection fraction, and chest radiograph reveals a pleural effusion. What type of effusion is most likely?

34. What condition classically presents with a harsh barking cough and stridor?

35. A 69-year-old man who recently retired from a life-long mining career with exposure to asbestos presents to the clinic with insidious onset of dyspnea, non-pleuritic chest pain, and weight loss. He denies history of tobacco use. Chest radiograph reveals pleural effusion. Thoracentesis is performed, and malignant cells are identified. What is the most likely diagnosis?

36. What home therapy is commonly recommended for mucous clearance in patients with cystic fibrosis and includes techniques such as postural drainage and percussion?

37. A 42-year-old woman presents to the clinic with slow onset of fatigue and mild dyspnea. A couple of months ago, red tender lumps developed on the shins, which resolved without treatment. Chest radiograph reveals hilar lymphadenopathy. Angiotensin-converting enzyme levels are elevated and noncaseating granulomas are identified on histology. What is the initial class of medication that may be recommended?

38. Which ribs are vertebrochondral?

39. A thin, 74-year-old man with a 40-pack year history of tobacco use presents to the clinic with chronic cough and dyspnea after not seeing a medical provider for over a decade. Physical exam reveals decreased breath sounds and difficulty breathing through pursed lips. What is the presumptive diagnosis?

40. What class of medication most commonly causes a drug-induced cough?

(See answers next page.)

33. Transudative effusion

The clinical vignette supports the diagnosis of congestive heart failure (CHF). The most common causes of transudative effusion include CHF and cirrhosis; whereas, exudative effusions are infection and malignancy.

Blueprint Task: Using Diagnostic and Laboratory Studies
Cognitive Level: Analyze

34. Croup (viral laryngotracheobronchitis)

Blueprint Task: History Taking and Performing Physical Examination
Cognitive Level: Recall

35. Malignant mesothelioma

Occupational hazards must be assessed to identify risk for asbestosis-related cancer.

Blueprint Task: Formulating Most Likely Diagnosis
Cognitive Level: Apply

36. Chest physiotherapy

Blueprint Task: Health Maintenance, Patient Education, and Preventive Measures
Cognitive Level: Recall

37. Corticosteroids

The clinical vignette supports the diagnosis of sarcoidosis. The lower extremity findings are consistent with erythema nodosum. If the patient experiences no improvement with corticosteroids, immunomodulatory agents may be recommended.

Blueprint Task: Pharmaceutical Therapeutics
Cognitive Level: Analyze

38. 8th, 9th, and 10th

Blueprint Task: Applying Basic Scientific Concepts
Cognitive Level: Recall

39. Emphysema

Patients with emphysema and respiratory compromise typically present with pink skin, rather than cyanotic. As such, they have previously been described as "pink puffers".

Blueprint Task: Formulating Most Likely Diagnosis
Cognitive Level: Apply

40. Angiotensin-converting enzyme (ACE) inhibitor

Blueprint Task: Pharmaceutical Therapeutics
Cognitive Level: Recall

41. Total lung capacity (TLC) is calculated by adding vital capacity (VC) to what other measurement?

42. What portable device is recommended for tracking asthma control and may detect an asthma exacerbation?

43. A healthy 23-year-old man with incomplete immunization status presents to the clinic with persistent cough. Last week he had nasal congestion, mild cough, and malaise. Coughing attacks have intensified leading to posttussive emesis. Other members of his household have similar symptoms. What is the first-line medication class recommended for the presumptive diagnosis?

44. Optimal needle decompression placement for tension pneumothorax should be performed either at the second intercostal space, midclavicular line, or at what other anatomical landmark?

45. A 3-year-old girl presents to the clinic with a 2-day history of cough and is diagnosed with a viral upper respiratory infection. She remains playful and appears well. The mother inquiries about over-the-counter (OTC) cough medicine for nighttime coughing. What is the recommendation regarding the use of these medications in this age group?

46. A patient with a history of asthma presents to the emergency department in respiratory distress with blue discoloration of the skin. What term describes the discoloration?

47. A healthy 40-year-old man, with no history of prior headaches, presents to the emergency department with a dull headache and mild nausea since this morning. The headache has improved since leaving his house. He recently began using a propane space heater. Physical exam reveals no focal neurologic deficits or significant abnormalities. What laboratory test will confirm the presumptive diagnosis?

48. What is the most common cause of hemoptysis presenting to an outpatient clinic?

49. What prompt procedure should be performed, along with empiric antibiotics, in the management of an empyema?

(*See answers next page.*)

41. Residual volume (RV)

Vital capacity measurement is the total of inspiratory reserve volume, tidal volume, and expiratory reserve volume. Residual volume must be determined to calculate total lung capacity. VC + RV = TLC.

Blueprint Task: Using Diagnostic and Laboratory Studies
Cognitive Level: Apply

42. Peak flow meter

Blueprint Task: Health Maintenance, Patient Education, and Preventive Measures
Cognitive Level: Recall

43. Macrolide

The clinical vignette supports the diagnosis of pertussis. Pertussis should be considered in patients with persistent cough lasting more than 2 weeks.

Blueprint Task: Pharmaceutical Therapeutics
Cognitive Level: Analyze

44. Fourth intercostal space, anterior axillary line

Blueprint Task: Clinical Intervention
Cognitive Level: Recall

45. OTC cough medications are not recommended

OTC cold and cough medications do not provide significant benefits and have the potential for serious risk in younger children. Reassurance, cool mist humidification, rest, and fluids are recommended.

Blueprint Task: Health Maintenance, Patient Education, and Preventive Measures
Cognitive Level: Apply

46. Cyanosis

Blueprint Task: History Taking and Performing Physical Examination
Cognitive Level: Recall

47. Carboxyhemoglobin saturation

The presumptive diagnosis is carbon monoxide exposure, and elevated carboxyhemoglobin would confirm the diagnosis.

Blueprint Task: Using Diagnostic and Laboratory Studies
Cognitive Level: Analyze

48. Pulmonary infection

Blueprint Task: History Taking and Performing Physical Examination
Cognitive Level: Recall

49. Drainage

Blueprint Task: Clinical Intervention
Cognitive Level: Recall

50. What antibiotic, commonly used for urinary tract infections, is associated with acute and chronic pulmonary hypersensitivity reactions?

51. What criteria are helpful in differentiating an exudative from a transudative pleural effusion by utilizing ratios of lactate dehydrogenase and protein levels in the pleural fluid versus serum?

52. A 47-year-old woman underwent a small bowel resection 2 days ago. Vital signs were stable both prior to and during the procedure. Physical exam reveals mild tachypnea and tachycardia with hypoxemia. Chest radiograph reveals bilateral, linear, increased density with displacement of the interlobar fissures. What post-surgical complication is described?

53. What pulmonary finding describes low-pitched lung sounds that classically resolve with a cough?

54. A tall, thin 22-year-old man with a history of tobacco use presents to the emergency department with right-sided chest pain and shortness of breath that began abruptly 4 hours ago. Physical exam reveals tachycardia and decreased right-sided breath sounds. Chest radiograph is shown below. What is the most likely diagnosis?

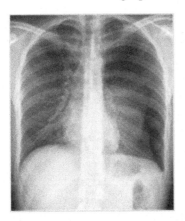

55. What abnormal type of respiration may present with heart failure and is characterized by a pattern of hypoventilation, apnea, and hyperventilation?

56. Metastatic pulmonary disease is suspected in a patient with breast cancer. Chest radiograph reveals multiple nodules in the periphery of the lung fields bilaterally. What is the next step in the imaging evaluation?

57. What tool is recommended by the Global Initiative for Chronic Obstructive Lung Disease (GOLD) to assess patient symptoms and determine the risk for worsening chronic obstructive lung disease (COPD)?

58. A 23-year-old woman with asthma presents to the clinic with rhinorrhea, sore throat, cough, diffuse myalgia, and fever since yesterday. She has not been vaccinated since childhood. Pulmonary exam is unremarkable, and COVID testing is negative. What class of medication may speed resolution of symptoms if initiated within 48 hours of symptom onset?

(*See answers next page.*)

50. Nitrofurantoin

Nitrofurantoin-induced pulmonary injury causes symptoms such as dyspnea and cough lasting days to months after medication use.
Blueprint Task: *Pharmaceutical Therapeutics*
Cognitive Level: *Apply*

51. Light's criteria

Blueprint Task: *Applying Basic Scientific Concepts*
Cognitive Level: *Recall*

52. Atelectasis

Atelectasis may occur post-operatively, typically from lack of clearance of secretions while under general anesthesia and due to postoperative pain restricting ventilation.
Blueprint Task: *Formulating Most Likely Diagnosis*
Cognitive Level: *Apply*

53. Rhonchi

Blueprint Task: *History Taking and Performing Physical Examination*
Cognitive Level: *Recall*

54. Pneumothorax

The clinical vignette and chest radiograph support the diagnosis of pneumothorax.
Blueprint Task: *Formulating Most Likely Diagnosis*
Cognitive Level: *Analyze*

55. Cheyne Stokes breathing

Blueprint Task: *History Taking and Performing Physical Examination*
Cognitive Level: *Recall*

56. CT of chest

Blueprint Task: *Using Diagnostic and Laboratory Studies*
Cognitive Level: *Recall*

57. Refined ABCD Assessment Tool for COPD

Blueprint Task: *Applying Basic Scientific Concepts*
Cognitive Level: *Recall*

58. Neuraminidase inhibitors

The clinical vignette supports an early presentation of influenza in a high-risk patient due to the history of asthma. The most commonly used neuraminidase inhibitor is oseltamivir.
Blueprint Task: *Pharmaceutical Therapeutics*
Cognitive Level: *Analyze*

59. What abnormal physical exam finding presents as irregular angles between the nail and the nail folds and is associated with chronic pulmonary disease?

60. A 24-year-old man is involved in a high-speed motor vehicle accident and suffered significant blunt chest wall trauma after being ejected from the vehicle. Chest radiographs are negative. 24-hours following admission to the hospital, he becomes hypoxic, and a repeat chest radiograph reveals a unilateral, non-lobar opacity of the right lung parenchyma. What is the most likely diagnosis?

61. A 20-year-old man has severe asthma uncontrolled with high-dose corticosteroids. What injectable recombinant antibody therapy that binds to circulating IgE may be recommended in this patient?

62. A 35-year-old man was rescued after being trapped in a house fire. He sustained burns to the face and neck with black discoloration around the nostrils. He developed severe dyspnea. What initial intervention is necessary for airway protection?

63. What treatment is used in conditions such as decompression sickness by delivering 100% oxygen inside a pressurized chamber?

64. What is the most common benign tumor presenting as a solitary pulmonary nodule?

65. A toddler presents to the emergency department with his father who reports that while eating a hot dog, his son abruptly began gagging and has not been breathing normally. Physical exam reveals tachypnea and coughing. Upon auscultation, wheezing and decreased breath sounds are noted. What procedure is diagnostic and therapeutic for the presumptive diagnosis?

66. A patient with metastatic lung cancer presents with dyspnea. Chest radiography shows a right elevated hemidiaphragm. What is the presumptive diagnosis?

67. A 29-year-old man experiences a near-drowning event when learning to surf. Within 24 hours, he develops confusion and profound dyspnea with tachypnea and tachycardia. What is the presumptive diagnosis based on the following image?

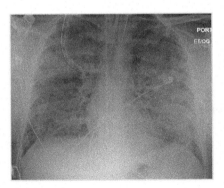

(*See answers next page.*)

59. Digital clubbing
Blueprint Task: History Taking and Performing Physical Examination
Cognitive Level: Recall

60. Pulmonary contusion
Pulmonary contusion is a common injury following blunt thoracic trauma and may take 24-48 hours to be observable on imaging.
Blueprint Task: Using Diagnostic and Laboratory Studies
Cognitive Level: Apply

61. Omalizumab
Blueprint Task: Pharmaceutical Therapeutics
Cognitive Level: Recall

62. Endotracheal intubation
The clinical vignette supports the diagnosis of thermal inhalation injury. Airway edema may quickly develop, leading to loss of airway.
Blueprint Task: Clinical Intervention
Cognitive Level: Apply

63. Hyperbaric oxygen therapy
Blueprint Task: Pharmaceutical Therapeutics
Cognitive Level: Recall

64. Hamartoma
Blueprint Task: Applying Basic Scientific Concepts
Cognitive Level: Recall

65. Rigid bronchoscopy with foreign body removal
The clinical vignette supports the diagnosis of partial airway obstruction secondary to foreign body aspiration. A rigid bronchoscopy enables visualization of the foreign body for removal.
Blueprint Task: Clinical Intervention
Cognitive Level: Analyze

66. Phrenic nerve compression
Blueprint Task: Formulating Most Likely Diagnosis
Cognitive Level: Recall

67. Acute respiratory distress syndrome (ARDS)
ARDS is characterized by acute respiratory distress progressing to respiratory failure and may be caused by a variety of factors such as pulmonary trauma, sepsis, or drug overdose.
Blueprint Task: Formulating Most Likely Diagnosis
Cognitive Level: Analyze

68. What would be the minimum respiratory rate for tachypnea in a toddler?

69. A 73-year-old man who worked in construction installing insulation for 45 years presents for evaluation of dyspnea on exertion. Chest radiograph reveals opacities in the lower lung fields with "ground-glass" changes bilaterally. What is the most likely diagnosis associated with his occupational exposures?

70. A 65-year-old man with a history of lung cancer presents to the clinic with worsening shortness of breath, cough, and facial swelling. Physical exam reveals bilateral arm edema, plethora, and jugular venous distension. Chest radiographs are concerning for a tumor invading the mediastinum. What is the most likely diagnosis?

71. What is a quick, noninvasive method of measuring arterial oxygen saturation?

72. A patient presents to the emergency department with severe shortness of breath secondary to an asthma exacerbation. She is hypoxic, tachycardic, and tachypneic with accessory muscle use. Signs and symptoms do not improve with oxygen, bronchodilators, and corticosteroids. What diagnosis would best characterize her current clinical presentation?

73. Prolonged immobility, such as extensive air travel, significantly increases the risk of what pulmonary condition in an otherwise healthy patient?

74. What blood test may aid in the diagnosis of venous thromboembolism and pulmonary embolism?

75. The mother of a 3-year-old child with asthma requests the intranasal live attenuated influenza vaccine (LAIV) rather than the injection of the inactivated influenza vaccine (IIV). What is the best patient education to provide regarding this request?

76. What device is recommended with a metered-dose inhaler to improve inhaled medication delivery and decrease deposition in the mouth and pharynx?

(See answers next page.)

68. >40 breaths/minute
Blueprint Task: History Taking and Performing Physical Examination
Cognitive Level: Recall

69. Asbestosis
The clinical vignette describes classic early symptoms and radiographic findings in a patient exposed to asbestos. Examples of occupational exposures include construction, shipbuilding, milling, or mining.
Blueprint Task: Using Diagnostic and Laboratory Studies
Cognitive Level: Apply

70. Superior vena cava (SVC) syndrome
Symptoms and signs demonstrated in the clinical vignette are caused by obstruction of blood flow through the SVC. The most common malignant cause of SVC is lung cancer or lymphoma.
Blueprint Task: Formulating Most Likely Diagnosis
Cognitive Level: Analyze

71. Pulse oximetry
Blueprint Task: History Taking and Performing Physical Examination
Cognitive Level: Recall

72. Status asthmaticus
Patients with status asthmaticus may require additional treatment such as magnesium.
Blueprint Task: Formulating Most Likely Diagnosis
Cognitive Level: Apply

73. Pulmonary embolism
Prolonged immobility increases risk of development for deep vein thrombosis (DVT), which may lead to pulmonary embolism.
Blueprint Task: Health Maintenance, Patient Education, and Preventive Measures
Cognitive Level: Apply

74. D-dimer assay
Blueprint Task: Applying Basic Scientific Concepts
Cognitive Level: Recall

75. LAIV would not be recommended
Based on the clinical vignette, IIV is typically recommended rather than LAIV since LAIV may be associated with asthma exacerbations in young children.
Blueprint Task: Health Maintenance, Patient Education, and Preventive Measures
Cognitive Level: Apply

76. Inhalation chamber (spacer)
Blueprint Task: Clinical Intervention
Cognitive Level: Recall

77. A 50-year-old man sustained a penetrating chest wall injury and presents with chest pain and dyspnea. Physical exam reveals tachycardia, hypotension, and decreased breath sounds. Chest radiograph is provided here. What is the most likely diagnosis?

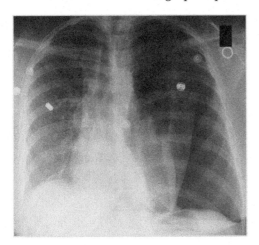

78. What breath sound creates a high-pitched, whistling quality caused by obstruction with airway resistance?

79. A 55-year-old man with severe alcoholism presents with fever, cough, and sputum production. Chest radiograph reveals a thick-walled cavity with an air-fluid level. What additional study would further evaluate the cavitation and help support the presumptive diagnosis?

80. A 28-year-old man presents to the emergency department by ambulance after a motorcycle accident. He is hypoxic with severe dyspnea and paradoxical chest movements. Chest radiograph reveals nine adjacent rib fractures. What is the presumptive diagnosis?

81. What vaccination significantly decreased cases of epiglottitis in children?

82. What color-based protocol uses three zones to identify worsening asthma symptoms and outlines management recommendations?

83. A 70-year-old woman presents to the clinic with a dry cough, fever, fatigue, and shortness of breath for 2 days. Prior to developing these symptoms, she lost her taste and smell. She recently attended a wedding with close family members, and many of them have similar symptoms of varying degrees. What is the most likely diagnosis?

84. What chest wall deformity is caused by chronically overinflated lungs and is associated with long-standing obstructive lung disease?

85. What medication is most likely to elicit a drug allergy?

(See answers next page.)

77. Tension pneumothorax

Potential causes of tension pneumothorax include trauma, infection, and mechanical ventilation.

Blueprint Task: *Formulating Most Likely Diagnosis*
Cognitive Level: *Apply*

78. Wheeze

Blueprint Task: *History Taking and Performing Physical Examination*
Cognitive Level: *Recall*

79. CT of chest

The clinical vignette supports the diagnosis of pulmonary abscess. Alcoholism increases the risk of aspiration leading to pulmonary abscess.

Blueprint Task: *Using Diagnostic and Laboratory Studies*
Cognitive Level: *Analyze*

80. Flail chest

Flail chest is defined by fractures of ≥3 contiguous ribs. Early intubation and mechanical ventilation are recommended for severe flail chest.

Blueprint Task: *Formulating Most Likely Diagnosis*
Cognitive Level: *Apply*

81. *Haemophilus influenzae* type b (Hib) vaccine

Blueprint Task: *Applying Basic Scientific Concepts*
Cognitive Level: *Recall*

82. Asthma action plan

Blueprint Task: *Health Maintenance, Patient Education, and Preventive Measures*
Cognitive Level: *Recall*

83. Coronavirus disease 2019 (COVID-19)

COVID-19 is caused by SARS-CoV-2 virus and was declared a global pandemic in 2020. Many patients are asymptomatic. Anosmia and dysgeusia are important diagnostic features that typically present early in the clinical presentation. Main clinical findings include fever, cough, and dyspnea. Additional symptoms may include myalgias, fatigue, headaches, or gastrointestinal complaints.

Blueprint Task: *Formulating Most Likely Diagnosis*
Cognitive Level: *Apply*

84. Barrel chest

Blueprint Task: *History Taking and Performing Physical Examination*
Cognitive Level: *Recall*

85. Penicillin

Blueprint Task: *Pharmaceutical Therapeutics*
Cognitive Level: *Recall*

86. A 13-year-old boy has a history of chronic sinusitis and malabsorption. During acute respiratory illnesses, he frequently develops cough, thick mucus, and dyspnea. What is the most likely chronic condition that is an autosomal recessive disorder affecting multiple organs?

87. What nebulized medication may be used in combination with corticosteroids for the treatment of severe croup?

88. Catamenial asthma is characterized by what hormonally mediated process?

89. A 64-year-old woman with chronic obstructive pulmonary disease (COPD) presents to the emergency department with worsening dyspnea over the past few days. Oxygen saturation is 90% on room air. The arterial blood gas (ABG) reveals a pH of 7.29, $PaCO_2$ of 60 mmHg, HCO_3 of 29 mmol/L, and PaO_2 of 75 mmHg. What is the primary acid-base disorder?

90. What disorder typically presents with chronic productive cough and wheezing characterized by airway dilation and bronchial wall thickening?

91. What is the gold standard to diagnose and quantify the severity of pulmonary hypertension?

92. A 74-year-old man with a history of lung cancer presents to the clinic for eyelid drooping and changes in perspiration. Physical exam reveals unequal pupil size with slight drooping of the right eyelid. What syndrome is associated with this clinical presentation?

93. Following a positive AFB and NAA, what test provides a definitive diagnosis of pulmonary tuberculosis?

94. During cancer staging, what does the M represent in TNM?

95. A 72-year-old man with a long-standing history of tobacco use is found to have an enlarging solitary pulmonary nodule on chest radiographs. He denies prior advanced imaging. What imaging study should be ordered next to further evaluate the nodule?

(See answers next page.)

86. Cystic fibrosis (CF)
CF may affect lungs, sinuses, pancreas, liver, and intestines.
Blueprint Task: Formulating Most Likely Diagnosis
Cognitive Level: Apply

87. Epinephrine
Blueprint Task: Clinical Intervention
Cognitive Level: Recall

88. Menstrual cycle
Blueprint Task: History Taking and Performing Physical Examination
Cognitive Level: Recall

89. Respiratory acidosis
The ABG interpretation represents primary respiratory acidosis with compensatory metabolic alkalosis resulting from pulmonary retention and impaired excretion of carbon dioxide.
Blueprint Task: Using Diagnostic and Laboratory Studies
Cognitive Level: Analyze

90. Bronchiectasis
Blueprint Task: Formulating Most Likely Diagnosis
Cognitive Level: Recall

91. Right-sided cardiac catheterization
Blueprint Task: Clinical Intervention
Cognitive Level: Recall

92. Horner syndrome
Horner syndrome consists of ipsilateral ptosis, miosis, and anhidrosis.
Blueprint Task: History Taking and Performing Physical Examination
Cognitive Level: Apply

93. Sputum culture
Blueprint Task: Using Diagnostic and Laboratory Studies
Cognitive Level: Recall

94. Metastasis
Blueprint Task: Health Maintenance, Patient Education, and Preventive Measures
Cognitive Level: Recall

95. CT of chest
The CT will further delineate tumor location, size, density, calcification, and other key characteristics to guide the differential diagnosis and management plan.
Blueprint Task: Clinical Intervention
Cognitive Level: Apply

Renal System

1. A 40-year-old patient presents to the clinic with dysuria, flank pain, fever, and nausea increasing over the last 2 days. On physical exam, kidneys are tender with deep palpation. White blood cell casts are present on urinalysis. What specialized physical exam technique would further support the presumptive diagnosis?

2. A 28-year-old man presents to the clinic with an episode of gross hematuria. He is without irritative voiding symptoms. He developed cold symptoms a day or two ago. Urinalysis reveals hematuria and proteinuria <3 g/day. What is the presumptive diagnosis?

3. A 67-year-old patient presents to the clinic for follow-up of type 2 diabetes, chronic kidney disease stage 4, and cirrhosis. Chronic medications include lisinopril and spironolactone. What electrolyte should be monitored closely in this patient?

4. What malignancy is a patient with a horseshoe kidney at an increased risk for developing?

5. Aside from iron replacement, what pharmaceutical therapy may be appropriate in patients with anemia of chronic kidney disease?

6. At what stage of chronic kidney disease (CKD) should patients be referred to a nephrologist for consideration of renal replacement therapy?

7. A 45-year-old man presents to the clinic with chronic bloody nasal discharge, cough, dyspnea, and hematuria. A chest radiograph reveals lung infiltrates and cavitations. Serology reveals + C-ANCA. What is the most likely diagnosis?

1. Costovertebral angle (CVA) tenderness
The clinical vignette supports the diagnosis of pyelonephritis. CVA tenderness is assessed with fist percussion along the bilateral flanks.
Blueprint Task: History Taking and Performing Physical Examination
Cognitive Level: Analyze

2. IgA nephropathy
The clinical vignette supports the diagnosis of IgA nephropathy. IgA nephropathy presents in the nephritic spectrum of renal diseases with gross hematuria 1–2 days following the onset of an upper respiratory infection.
Blueprint Task: Formulating Most Likely Diagnosis
Cognitive Level: Apply

3. Potassium
Concomitant use of angiotensin-converting enzyme (ACE) inhibitor, angiotensin receptor blocker (ARB), and aldosterone antagonists may precipitate hyperkalemia.
Blueprint Task: Pharmaceutical Therapeutics
Cognitive Level: Apply

4. Wilms tumor
Blueprint Task: Applying Basic Scientific Concepts
Cognitive Level: Recall

5. Erythropoiesis-stimulating agents
Anemia of chronic kidney disease can lead to a decrease in erythropoietin production. Erythropoiesis-stimulating agents (i.e., recombinant human erythropoietin) stimulate RBC production.
Blueprint Task: Clinical Intervention
Cognitive Level: Apply

6. Late-stage CKD 3
Blueprint Task: Health Maintenance, Patient Education, and Preventive Measures
Cognitive Level: Recall

7. Granulomatosis with polyangiitis (GPA)
The clinical vignette supports the diagnosis of GPA, formerly known as Wegener granulomatosis, an anti-neutrophil cytoplasmic autoantibody (ANCA) associated vasculitis. GPA causes necrotizing granulomatous inflammation (commonly affecting the respiratory tract) and leads to rapidly progressive glomerulonephritis.
Blueprint Task: Formulating Most Likely Diagnosis
Cognitive Level: Analyze

8. What electrocardiogram (ECG) abnormality is most commonly associated with hypocalcemia?

9. A 3-year-old boy presents to the clinic with sudden weight gain. He is recovering from a viral upper respiratory infection and is found to have hypoalbuminemia and proteinuria (>3.5 g/day) with a bland urinary sediment. What is the most likely physical exam finding based on the presumptive diagnosis?

10. A 49-year-old man with hyperlipidemia, 40-pack-year tobacco history, and newly diagnosed type 2 diabetes has an episode of acute kidney injury following the initiation of lisinopril. The physical exam reveals an abdominal bruit. Abdominal ultrasound reveals asymmetric kidney size. What is the presumptive diagnosis?

11. Chronic kidney disease leading to secondary hyperparathyroidism and metabolic bone disease requires management of hypocalcemia and hypovitaminosis D. What other electrolyte needs to be corrected in this setting?

12. What is the first-line pharmacologic therapy utilized for patients with pyelonephritis in the outpatient setting?

13. A patient presents with hypotension after 3 days of intractable nausea and vomiting. Activation of the renin-angiotensin-aldosterone system (RAAS) may result in sodium and water retention and excretion of what electrolyte?

14. A 59-year-old man presents to the clinic with flank pain radiating to the groin and decreased urine output. A BMP reveals a BUN of 28 mg/dL and creatinine of 1.5 mg/dL. Renal ultrasound demonstrates dilated renal calyces. What clinical intervention is necessary to prevent progressive damage of renal parenchyma?

(*See answers next page.*)

8. QT prolongation
Blueprint Task: Using Diagnostic and Laboratory Studies
Cognitive Level: Recall

9. Edema
The clinical vignette supports nephrotic syndrome attributed to minimal change disease (MCD). MCD is one of the most common causes of nephrotic syndrome in children and is often preceded by a viral infection.
Blueprint Task: History Taking and Performing Physical Examination
Cognitive Level: Analyze

10. Renal artery stenosis
Renal artery stenosis accounts for the majority of renal vascular disease and often presents with acute kidney injury upon starting angiotensin-converting enzyme (ACE) inhibitor or angiotensin receptor blocker (ARB) therapy.
Blueprint Task: Formulating Most Likely Diagnosis
Cognitive Level: Analyze

11. Phosphorus
Hyperphosphatemia from chronic kidney disease can contribute to secondary hyperparathyroidism. Control of hyperphosphatemia via dietary phosphorus restriction and phosphate binders may help prevent worsening metabolic bone disease.
Blueprint Task: Health Maintenance, Patient Education, and Preventive Measures
Cognitive Level: Apply

12. Fluoroquinolones
Blueprint Task: Pharmaceutical Therapeutics
Cognitive Level: Recall

13. Potassium
The RAAS is a complex pathway that is activated in the setting of low blood pressure or ineffective circulating volume.
Blueprint Task: Applying Basic Scientific Concepts
Cognitive Level: Apply

14. Relieve obstruction
The patient is presenting with hydronephrosis, most likely secondary to a ureteral stone. Relief of obstruction is necessary to prevent tubular atrophy, interstitial fibrosis, renal injury, and other complications.
Blueprint Task: Clinical Intervention
Cognitive Level: Analyze

15. Slowing the progression of diabetic nephropathy requires maintaining optimal blood pressure and controlling what laboratory measurement?

16. A 38-year-old woman with severe anxiety presents to the emergency department hyperventilating and reports feeling lightheaded with perioral numbness. What acid–base disorder is most likely based on her symptoms?

17. What is the classic triad of signs and symptoms for renal carcinoma?

18. A patient with an obstructed kidney stone is placed on ciprofloxacin. What black-box warning is associated with this medication?

19. A 35-year-old healthy woman's recent laboratory evaluation reveals a potassium of 5.9 mEq/L. She is asymptomatic and takes no medications. What is the most appropriate next step in the work-up of this patient?

20. What is the target blood pressure goal in patients with chronic kidney disease with proteinuria?

21. A 68-year-old woman with end-stage renal disease missed multiple hemodialysis sessions. She presents to the emergency department with weight gain and edema. Labs demonstrate hyperkalemia and hyperphosphatemia. The ABG reveals a pH of 7.10, HCO_3 12 mmol/L, and pCO_2 32 mm Hg with an anion gap of 20 mEq/L. What is the most likely acid-base disorder?

(See answers next page.)

15. Blood glucose

Diabetic nephropathy is the most common cause of end-stage renal disease. Intensive blood glucose and blood pressure control are imperative.

Blueprint Task: Health Maintenance, Patient Education, and Preventive Measures
Cognitive Level: Apply

16. Respiratory alkalosis

Hyperventilation results in excessive elimination of CO_2 from the lungs and contributes to respiratory alkalosis. It may be caused by conditions such as anxiety, high altitude, and hypoxia.

Blueprint Task: Formulating Most Likely Diagnosis
Cognitive Level: Analyze

17. Hematuria, flank pain, and flank mass

Blueprint Task: Applying Basic Scientific Concepts
Cognitive Level: Recall

18. Risk of tendinitis and tendon rupture

Fluoroquinolones may lead to tendinitis and tendon rupture, most commonly affecting the Achilles tendon.

Blueprint Task: Pharmaceutical Therapeutics
Cognitive Level: Apply

19. Repeat a potassium level

The clinical vignette supports the diagnosis of pseudohyperkalemia. In the absence of kidney disease or high-risk medications causing hyperkalemia, a repeat lab test should be done. Pseudohyperkalemia is a laboratory artifact that may result from poor venipuncture technique.

Blueprint Task: Clinical Intervention
Cognitive Level: Analyze

20. <130/80 mm Hg

Blueprint Task: Health Maintenance, Patient Education, and Preventive Measures
Cognitive Level: Recall

21. Metabolic acidosis

Metabolic acidosis with an elevated anion gap can be seen in patients with renal failure. Treatment of the underlying disorder is necessary.

Blueprint Task: Formulating Most Likely Diagnosis
Cognitive Level: Analyze

22. A 40-year-old man with a history of hypertension and a family history of "kidney problems" presents as a new patient to the clinic. He reports intermittent abdominal and flank pain. Physical exam reveals elevated blood pressure and large, palpable kidneys. Labs reveal hematuria. What is the initial imaging of choice to evaluate for the presumptive diagnosis?

23. Poststreptococcal glomerulonephritis typically occurs days to weeks after a streptococcal infection. What are the two most common anatomic sites that the infection originates?

24. A 77-year-old woman with a history of hypertension presents to the emergency department with shortness of breath and weight gain over the past few days. She complains of waking up at night gasping for air and sleeping propped up with multiple pillows. On physical exam, she has pulmonary rales, jugular venous distention, and lower extremity edema. Labs reveal a Na of 126 mEq/L, BUN 38 mg/dL, and Cr 1.6 mg/dL. What type of kidney injury is most likely based on the presumptive diagnosis?

25. What two classes of medications are most appropriate for the treatment of proteinuria to prevent the progression of kidney disease and reduce cardiovascular disease risk?

26. Slow cautious correction of acute hyponatremia is necessary to prevent what complication?

27. A 10-year-old boy presents to the clinic with dark, cola-colored urine over the last 1–2 days. He has no dysuria or fever, but his mother reports that her son's face appears to be swollen. The patient had a recent sore throat that resolved without treatment. Laboratory evaluation reveals red blood cell casts and a positive ASO titer. What is the most likely diagnosis?

28. In a patient with edema, hyperlipidemia, and proteinuria >3.5 g/day, what pharmacologic therapy may be recommended due to the urinary losses of antithrombin, protein C, and protein S?

(See answers next page.)

22. Ultrasound

The clinical vignette supports the diagnosis of autosomal dominant polycystic kidney disease. Typical findings on ultrasound include enlarged kidneys with multiple cysts.

Blueprint Task: Using Diagnostic and Laboratory Studies
Cognitive Level: Analyze

23. Pharynx and skin

Blueprint Task: History Taking and Performing Physical Examination
Cognitive Level: Recall

24. Prerenal acute kidney injury (AKI)

The clinical vignette supports the diagnosis of congestive heart failure, leading to prerenal AKI caused by ineffective circulating volume and renal hypoperfusion. Prerenal AKI is associated with a Bun/Cr ratio >20:1. Prolonged hypoperfusion may lead to intrinsic renal disease.

Blueprint Task: Using Diagnostic and Laboratory Studies
Cognitive Level: Analyze

25. Angiotensin-converting enzyme (ACE) inhibitor and angiotensin receptor blocker (ARB)

Blueprint Task: Health Maintenance, Patient Education, and Preventive Measures
Cognitive Level: Recall

26. Osmotic demyelination syndrome (ODS)

Rapid correction of sodium may increase the risk for osmotic demyelination syndrome, formerly termed central pontine myelinolysis.

Blueprint Task: Clinical Intervention
Cognitive Level: Apply

27. Poststreptococcal glomerulonephritis

Poststreptococcal glomerulonephritis presents in the nephritic spectrum and is often preceded by a recent pharyngitis or impetigo infection.

Blueprint Task: Formulating Most Likely Diagnosis
Cognitive Level: Apply

28. Anticoagulation

The clinical vignette supports nephrotic syndrome, which increases the risk of hypercoagulability. Anticoagulation therapy may not be utilized in all patients. Lipid-lowering therapy may also be considered given the hyperlipidemia and risk of cardiovascular disease.

Blueprint Task: Pharmaceutical Therapeutics
Cognitive Level: Apply

29. What is a common, acute complication that can develop during hemodialysis as a result of rapid removal of fluid and shifts in plasma osmolality?

30. What vital sign would most likely be abnormal in a patient with autosomal dominant polycystic kidney disease?

31. A 30-year-old man with a history of tobacco use presents to the emergency department with cough, hemoptysis, and hematuria. Labs reveal a positive anti-GBM antibody. What is the most likely diagnosis?

32. What electrolyte should be monitored and replaced in patients with refractory hypokalemia and hypocalcemia?

33. A 78-year-old patient presents to the emergency department with perioral numbness and paresthesia of the fingers and toes. On physical exam, inflation of the blood pressure cuff to 20 mm Hg above the patient's systolic blood pressure for 3 minutes induces carpopedal spasms. What treatment is most appropriate given the presumptive diagnosis?

34. What two conditions most commonly cause chronic kidney disease?

35. A 78-year-old hospitalized patient currently on gentamicin therapy is found to have hyperkalemia, hyperphosphatemia, elevated BUN, and creatinine on morning labs. Urine microscopy reveals granular casts. What renal condition is most likely in this patient?

(See answers next page.)

29. Hypotension
Blueprint Task: Applying Basic Scientific Concepts
Cognitive Level: Recall

30. Blood pressure
Large palpable kidneys and hypertension are key features of polycystic kidney disease.
Blueprint Task: History Taking and Performing Physical Examination
Cognitive Level: Apply

31. Goodpasture syndrome
The clinical vignette supports the diagnosis of glomerulonephritis with pulmonary hemorrhage.
Blueprint Task: Formulating Most Likely Diagnosis
Cognitive Level: Apply

32. Magnesium
Hypomagnesemia may cause renal potassium wasting contributing to refractory hypokalemia. Hypomagnesemia may suppress parathyroid hormone release contributing to refractory hypocalcemia.
Blueprint Task: Clinical Intervention
Cognitive Level: Apply

33. Calcium gluconate
The clinical vignette supports the diagnosis of hypocalcemia with evidence of Trousseau sign. Treatment with calcium gluconate is appropriate for symptomatic hypocalcemia.
Blueprint Task: Pharmaceutical Therapeutics
Cognitive Level: Analyze

34. Diabetes and hypertension
Blueprint Task: Applying Basic Scientific Concepts
Cognitive Level: Recall

35. Acute tubular necrosis
Acute tubular necrosis can result from nephrotoxin exposure (e.g., aminoglycosides, IV contrast) and is most likely to cause intrinsic acute kidney injury with granular "muddy brown" casts.
Blueprint Task: Using Diagnostic and Laboratory Studies
Cognitive Level: Apply

36. A 6-year-old boy presents to the clinic for colicky abdominal discomfort and knee pain with a recent history of upper respiratory infection. Urinalysis reveals hematuria and red blood cell casts. What dermatologic finding is consistent with the presumptive diagnosis?

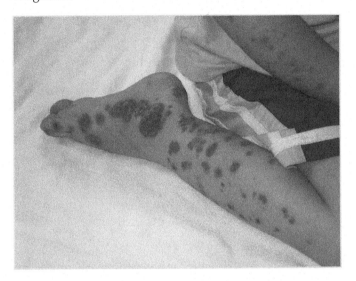

37. A 43-year-old woman presents to the clinic with hematuria. She has a systemic immune-mediated disorder associated with circulating anti-ds DNA antibodies. Labs reveal elevated creatinine, and urinalysis demonstrates proteinuria and red blood cell casts. What is the most likely diagnosis?

38. What clinical intervention is indicated for patients with refractory hyperkalemia or hyperphosphatemia, fluid overload unresponsive to diuresis, severe metabolic acidosis, or uremic symptoms?

39. Hypokalemia predisposes patients to toxicity of what medication and increases risk for arrhythmias?

40. What is the most reliable imaging test to confirm the diagnosis of ureterolithiasis?

41. A 67-year-old patient with type 2 diabetes, hypertension, hyperlipidemia, and end-stage renal disease presents to the emergency department with fatigue, weakness, nausea, and vomiting. A family member indicates that the patient has become progressively more irritable with memory impairment over the past few days. The patient has been missing dialysis appointments. What is the condition used to describe this constellation of symptoms?

42. What is the most common historical presentation of Wilms tumor that is often reported by parents?

(See answers next page.)

36. Palpable purpura rash

The clinical vignette supports the diagnosis of IgA vasculitis, formerly termed Henoch-Schönlein purpura. This condition commonly follows a viral illness and is defined by the classic tetrad of rash, arthralgia, abdominal pain, and renal disease.

Blueprint Task: History Taking and Performing Physical Examination
Cognitive Level: Analyze

37. Lupus nephritis

The clinical vignette supports the diagnosis of lupus nephritis. Anti-ds DNA antibodies are a common laboratory finding in patients with systemic lupus erythematosus.

Blueprint Task: Formulating Most Likely Diagnosis
Cognitive Level: Apply

38. Dialysis

Blueprint Task: Clinical Intervention
Cognitive Level: Recall

39. Digoxin

Potassium and digoxin competitively bind to the same cardiac site increasing the risk of digoxin toxicity and potentially leading to arrhythmias.

Blueprint Task: Pharmaceutical Therapeutics
Cognitive Level: Apply

40. Non-contrast computed tomography (CT)

Use of contrast may decrease visibility of a stone

Blueprint Task: Using Diagnostic and Laboratory Studies
Cognitive Level: Apply

41. Uremic syndrome

Uremic syndrome can develop with a significant decrease in GFR and results from the accumulation of metabolic waste products.

Blueprint Task: History Taking and Performing Physical Examination
Cognitive Level: Analyze

42. Asymptomatic abdominal mass

Blueprint Task: History Taking and Performing Physical Examination
Cognitive Level: Recall

43. A 54-year-old woman presents to the emergency department with intractable nausea, vomiting, and diarrhea. On physical exam, she is hypotensive and tachycardiac with decreased skin turgor and dry mucous membranes. Labs reveal a BUN of 42 mg/dL and creatinine of 1.8 mg/dL. Fractional excretion of sodium is <1%. What is the most appropriate initial intervention?

44. What over-the-counter analgesic/antipyretic class of medication should be avoided in patients with chronic kidney disease?

45. What renal disease, associated with bilaterally enlarged kidneys, may also be complicated by hepatic and pancreatic cysts?

46. A 22-year-old woman with a known history of vesicoureteral reflux is managed by her clinician for hypertension. What recurrent condition in childhood supports the clinical presentation?

47. A 33-year-old man with a history of Crohn disease presents to the emergency department with intractable vomiting and abdominal distention. Radiograph reveals dilated loops of bowel and air-fluid levels consistent with a small bowel obstruction. A nasogastric tube is placed to suction. Labs reveal hypokalemia and an ABG with a pH of 7.49, pCO_2 40 mm Hg, HCO_3 31 mmol/L. What primary acid–base disorder is most likely?

48. What would be considered a normal finding when palpating for the kidneys during a physical exam?

(See answers next page.)

43. Fluid resuscitation

The clinical vignette supports the diagnosis of prerenal acute kidney injury (AKI) secondary to dehydration. Dehydration is the most common cause of prerenal AKI. Fluid resuscitation is necessary to improve renal perfusion. Persistent hypoperfusion can lead to intrinsic renal disease.

Blueprint Task: *Clinical Intervention*
Cognitive Level: *Analyze*

44. Nonsteroidal anti-inflammatory drug (NSAID)

Blueprint Task: *Pharmaceutical Therapeutics*
Cognitive Level: *Recall*

45. Polycystic kidney disease

Polycystic kidney disease may present with extrarenal manifestations including hepatic and pancreatic cysts, valvular heart disease including mitral valve prolapse, and cerebral aneurysms.

Blueprint Task: *Formulating Most Likely Diagnosis*
Cognitive Level: *Apply*

46. Urinary tract infections

Vesicoureteral reflex results in the backflow of urine from the bladder into the upper urinary tract due to dysfunctional vesicoureteral sphincter. This reflux nephropathy can lead to fibrosis over time and contribute to hypertension.

Blueprint Task: *History Taking and Performing Physical Examination*
Cognitive Level: *Analyze*

47. Metabolic alkalosis

Metabolic alkalosis may result from vomiting and NG suction.

Blueprint Task: *Using Diagnostic and Laboratory Studies*
Cognitive Level: *Analyze*

48. Kidneys are non-palpable

The kidneys are typically non-palpable since they are retroperitoneal.

Blueprint Task: *History Taking and Performing Physical Examination*
Cognitive Level: *Apply*

Reproductive System (Male and Female)

1. During a pelvic exam, a healthy pregnant woman is found to have slight blue discoloration of the cervix. What is this sign?

2. A 42-year-old woman presents to the clinic because she discovered a nontender breast nodule. What first-line imaging study is recommended?

3. What is the most life-threatening complication of a vaginal birth following a previous cesarean birth (VBAC)?

4. A 38-year-old woman, who has not received prenatal care, presents to the emergency department in labor. During a vaginal delivery, the body of the newborn was unable to advance following delivery of the head. The head appears retracted against the perineum. What is the most likely cause of this presentation?

5. What is the typical recommended frequency of prenatal visits from 36 weeks' gestation until delivery?

6. A 35-year-old pregnant woman is found to have abnormal placement of the placenta over the internal cervical os. If this sonographic abnormality persists up until 37 weeks' gestation, what form of delivery is recommended?

7. A 22-year-old woman presents to the university health clinic requesting oral emergency contraception following a sexual assault that occurred 2 days ago. A combination hormonal contraception is prescribed. What pharmacologic class could be given prior to taking this medication to minimize common side effects?

8. In women >35 years of age seeking fertility, what laboratory test remains relatively consistent within the menstrual cycle and predicts ovarian reserve?

1. Chadwick sign

Blueprint Task: History Taking and Performing Physical Examination
Cognitive Level: Recall

2. Diagnostic mammogram

Mammograms are indicated for breast cancer assessment. Diagnostic mammograms are ordered for clinically abnormal breast exams. Screening mammogram is ordered for patients who are asymptomatic with normal breast exam.

Blueprint Task: Using Diagnostic and Laboratory Studies
Cognitive Level: Apply

3. Uterine rupture

Blueprint Task: Applying Basic Scientific Concepts
Cognitive Level: Recall

4. Shoulder dystocia

Shoulder dystocia is caused when the shoulders are unable to traverse the pelvis following delivery of the head. This presentation is critical to recognize early and requires emergent intervention. Common risk factors that may attribute to this birth complication include gestational diabetes, post-term pregnancy, prior shoulder dystocia, and macrosomia.

Blueprint Task: Formulating Most Likely Diagnosis
Cognitive Level: Analyze

5. Weekly

Blueprint Task: Health Maintenance, Patient Education, and Preventive Measures
Cognitive Level: Recall

6. Cesarean section

The clinical vignette supports the diagnosis of placenta previa. Common presentation is painless vaginal bleeding.

Blueprint Task: Clinical Intervention
Cognitive Level: Apply

7. Antiemetic

Oral emergency contraceptive regimens, particularly hormonal combinations, may cause nausea and vomiting. Antiemetic is typically prescribed 30–60 minutes prior to minimize these symptoms.

Blueprint Task: Pharmaceutical Therapeutics
Cognitive Level: Analyze

8. Anti-müllerian hormone (AMH)

Blueprint Task: Applying Basic Scientific Concepts
Cognitive Level: Recall

9. A 38-year-old woman who recently found out she was pregnant presents with acute severe lower right abdominal pain with vaginal bleeding. Bimanual exam reveals diffuse tenderness, exaggerated with cervical motion, and a questionable palpable right adnexal mass. What is the most likely diagnosis?

10. A 35-year-old nonlactating woman with a 15-pack year tobacco history presents to the clinic with a right-sided breast abscess. Incision and drainage are performed, and empiric antibiotics are prescribed. Once the abscess has resolved, what initial imaging study should be performed if concerned for underlying malignancy?

11. What is the initial recommended screening test for gestational diabetes mellitus (GDM) that is typically ordered for patients between 24 and 28 weeks' gestation?

12. Many women develop hyperpigmentation of the face during pregnancy that may fade after delivery. What initial patient education is recommended to avoid further hyperpigmentation associated with the presumptive diagnosis?

13. A 16-year-old girl presents to the clinic with a left breast mass. The breast exam reveals a 2-cm nontender, rubbery mass at 2 o'clock. What initial imaging study is preferred to further evaluate the presumptive diagnosis?

14. A multiparous woman presents for a well-woman visit. On physical exam, while bearing down, the posterior vaginal wall appears to bulge into the vagina. What is this finding?

15. A 37-year-old woman reports a positive home pregnancy test and recent development of nausea, vomiting, and irregular vaginal bleeding. On physical exam, the uterus is larger than expected. A quantitative serum beta-hCG is extremely high, and an ultrasound reveals no embryo. What is the most likely diagnosis?

(See answers next page.)

9. Ectopic pregnancy

Ectopic pregnancy may vary in presentation, with the most prominent symptoms being abdominal pain and vaginal bleeding. Referred pain may also present in the shoulder. Ruptured ectopic pregnancy may have the addition of syncope and shock.

Blueprint Task: Formulating Most Likely Diagnosis

Cognitive Level: Apply

10. Diagnostic mammogram

Breast abscesses are more commonly seen in nonlactating women who have a past medical history of tobacco use, elevated body mass index, or diabetes mellitus.

Blueprint Task: Clinical Intervention

Cognitive Level: Apply

11. Glucose tolerance test

Blueprint Task: Clinical Intervention

Cognitive Level: Recall

12. Sun protection

The clinical vignette supports the diagnosis of chloasma (also called melasma and the mask of pregnancy). Additional options for treatment, typically recommended postpartum, include topical skin lightening therapy and chemical peels.

Blueprint Task: Health Maintenance, Patient Education, and Preventive Measures

Cognitive Level: Analyze

13. Breast ultrasound

The clinical vignette supports the diagnosis of a fibroadenoma which is the most common breast mass in this age group. Ultrasound, rather than a mammogram, is the initial imaging study of choice due to the density of breast tissue in young women.

Blueprint Task: Using Diagnostic and Laboratory Studies

Cognitive Level: Analyze

14. Rectocele

Blueprint Task: History Taking and Performing Physical Examination

Cognitive Level: Recall

15. Hydatidiform mole

Hydatidiform mole is a type of gestational trophoblastic disease in which a tumor develops from the placenta without any fetal development. Ultrasound findings vary and may be classically described as a "snowstorm" appearance.

Blueprint Task: Formulating Most Likely Diagnosis

Cognitive Level: Apply

16. What is the most common medication used in the management of an ectopic pregnancy as an alternative to surgical intervention?

17. A 25-year-old woman presents to the emergency department following a sexual assault that occurred 24 hours prior. Besides performing a thorough history and physical exam, what other type of exam should be completed?

18. By what age, regardless of sexual intercourse, should a healthy patient receive her first Papanicolaou (PAP) test?

19. On pelvic exam, a 3-mm yellow raised lesion is visualized on the cervix. What is this benign finding?

20. In the acronym, TPAL, used to describe a woman's gynecologic history, P stands for premature deliveries, A for abortions, and L for living children. What does the T represent?

21. A healthy 25-year-old patient who is 20 weeks' gestation believes her immunizations are up to date; however, she has not received any immunizations since her last pregnancy 3 years ago. What two immunizations are recommended during the pregnancy?

22. A 28-year-old woman who is 36 weeks' gestation is found to have vaginal group B streptococcal (GBS) colonization. What therapy is recommended to provide during labor?

23. A 24-year-old woman presents to the clinic because she has not had a menstrual period in over 3 months. She does not have a previous history of irregular menses. What is the most important initial laboratory test?

24. What term identifies a vertical midline pigmentation extending from the suprapubic region to the umbilicus in a pregnant woman, as seen in the following image?

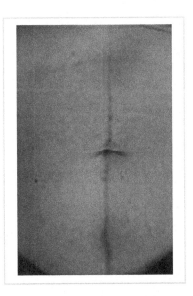

(See answers next page.)

16. Methotrexate

Blueprint Task: Pharmaceutical Therapeutics
Cognitive Level: Recall

17. Forensic exam

Forensic evidence kits allow for collection of physical evidence in cases of sexual assault. Typically, this evidence is collected within 72 hours of an assault though some hospital systems will extend this time to 96 hours.
Blueprint Task: Clinical Intervention
Cognitive Level: Apply

18. 21

Blueprint Task: Using Diagnostic and Laboratory Studies
Cognitive Level: Recall

19. Nabothian cyst

Nabothian cysts are typically asymptomatic and require no treatment.
Blueprint Task: History Taking and Performing Physical Examination
Cognitive Level: Apply

20. Term deliveries

Blueprint Task: Applying Basic Scientific Concepts
Cognitive Level: Recall

21. TDap and influenza

TDap is recommended during every pregnancy between 27 and 36 weeks' gestation. The influenza vaccine is recommended yearly and may be administered anytime during pregnancy.
Blueprint Task: Health Maintenance, Patient Education, and Preventive Measures
Cognitive Level: Apply

22. Penicillin G

Maternal colonization of GBS increases the risk for vertical transmission resulting in neonatal infection if prophylaxis is not administered. Neonatal GBS infections may lead to sepsis, pneumonia, or meningitis, which substantiates the critical need for screening during pregnancy.
Blueprint Task: Pharmaceutical Therapeutics
Cognitive Level: Apply

23. Beta-hCG

The clinical vignette supports the diagnosis of secondary amenorrhea, with the most common cause being pregnancy.
Blueprint Task: Using Diagnostic and Laboratory Studies
Cognitive Level: Apply

24. Linea nigra

Blueprint Task: History Taking and Performing Physical Examination
Cognitive Level: Recall

25. A patient who is 28 weeks' gestation presents to the emergency department with chest pain following a high-speed motor vehicle accident. She suffers cardiac arrest upon arrival. What clinical intervention should be considered at this time?

26. The expected date of delivery is often determined by subtracting 3 months from the date of the last menstrual period and then adding 7 days. What is this rule?

27. A 27-year-old woman presents to the emergency department with fever and severe pain in the right breast. She is 2 weeks postpartum and currently breastfeeding. On physical exam, she appears ill, and the right lower outer quadrant of her breast is red, swollen, and tender to palpation. What is the most likely causative organism associated with the presumptive diagnosis?

28. A 36-year-old postpartum woman presents to the clinic with continued milk discharge from both breasts despite never breastfeeding her baby. How long following childbirth would concern for galactorrhea be defined in this patient?

29. A 23-year-old woman with a history of migraines is placed on topiramate for headache prevention. She is sexually active, taking combined oral contraception, and does not wish to become pregnant. What patient education is recommended when taking both topiramate and an oral contraceptive pill (OCP)?

30. What is the most commonly used tumor marker in the evaluation of ovarian cancer?

31. A 32-year-old woman presents to the clinic with breast tenderness that worsens with menses. Physical exam reveals bilateral thickening of breast tissue without dominant mass. What dietary recommendation may decrease symptoms associated with the most likely diagnosis?

32. An 8-year-old girl presents with her mother to the clinic with concerns for early breast development. On physical exam, equal breast bud development is palpated with slightly elevated papillae. Genital exam reveals sparse, downy hair distribution. What classification would be commonly used to describe this patient's development?

(See answers next page.)

25. Emergent cesarean section

A resuscitative hysterotomy might be of benefit not only with delivery of the fetus but to improve cardiac function and ability to perform resuscitative efforts for the mother.

Blueprint Task: Clinical Intervention
Cognitive Level: Apply

26. Naegele's Rule

Blueprint Task: Applying Basic Scientific Concepts
Cognitive Level: Recall

27. *Staphylococcus aureus*

The clinical vignette supports the diagnosis of mastitis. The causative organism is typically introduced by a traumatized nipple during breastfeeding.

Blueprint Task: Formulating Most Likely Diagnosis
Cognitive Level: Analyze

28. 6 months

Galactorrhea is inappropriate milk discharge. Following childbirth, galactorrhea is defined as inappropriate milk discharge 6 months following termination of breastfeeding or 6 months postpartum in non-breastfeeding women.

Blueprint Task: Health Maintenance, Patient Education, and Preventive Measures
Cognitive Level: Apply

29. Additional contraception recommended

Some medications, such as some topiramate, may decrease the efficacy of OCP, warranting additional prevention.

Blueprint Task: Pharmaceutical Therapeutics
Cognitive Level: Apply

30. CA-125

Blueprint Task: Using Diagnostic and Laboratory Studies
Cognitive Level: Recall

31. Caffeine avoidance

The clinical vignette supports the diagnosis of fibrocystic breast changes, formerly called fibrocystic breast disease. Discontinuation of caffeine may decrease breast sensitivity but may not be effective in all patients. Supportive bras and analgesics can be beneficial.

Blueprint Task: Health Maintenance, Patient Education, and Preventive Measures
Cognitive Level: Analyze

32. Tanner stage II

Tanner sex maturity rating stages in females are based on characteristics of the breast and pubic hair development. Stage I is prepubertal, while stage V is the final stage and reflects adult formation.

Blueprint Task: History Taking and Performing Physical Examination
Cognitive Level: Analyze

33. A 36-year-old pregnant woman is brought by ambulance to the emergency department, actively seizing. Her husband indicates that she was being closely monitored for hypertension but has not been seen recently. Following administration of magnesium sulfate, what intervention is required to prevent further progression?

34. What nonsurgical, nonhormonal contraceptive method is most effective in pregnancy prevention?

35. A 38-year-old woman with a BMI of 33 kg/m^2 presents for a routine obstetric visit at 34 weeks' gestation. She is feeling well and reports no concerns. She has new-onset hypertension, and laboratory evaluation reveals proteinuria. What is the most likely diagnosis?

36. A 12-year-old boy presents to the clinic with tender thickening under both nipples that has been present for a few months. Physical exam reveals no nodularity, warmth, or other abnormality. What patient education should be provided given the presumptive diagnosis?

37. What is the average age range of menarche in the United States?

38. A 21-year-old woman with history of a previous sexually transmitted infection presents to the clinic with abnormal vaginal discharge, pelvic pain, and fever. During the bimanual exam, the patient experiences severe pain with cervical motion. What sign describes this abnormal physical exam finding?

39. How is the fern test used during pregnancy?

40. When does the second stage of labor begin?

41. During the third trimester, fetal position has consistently maintained buttocks downward, bilateral hip flexion, and knee extension with the feet near the head. What musculoskeletal condition is the infant at a higher risk for due to this positioning in utero that requires screening after birth?

(See answers next page.)

33. Urgent delivery of fetus

The clinical vignette supports the diagnosis of eclampsia. Emergent management is focused on the treatment of seizures and hypertension to stabilize the patient for delivery.

Blueprint Task: Clinical Intervention

Cognitive Level: Analyze

34. Copper intrauterine device (IUD)

Blueprint Task: Pharmaceutical Therapeutics

Cognitive Level: Recall

35. Preeclampsia

Risks for preeclampsia include factors such as advanced age, elevated BMI, and nulliparity.

Blueprint Task: Formulating Most Likely Diagnosis

Cognitive Level: Apply

36. Reassurance

The clinical vignette supports the diagnosis of physiologic gynecomastia, which is common in boys going through puberty and typically spontaneously resolves.

Blueprint Task: Health Maintenance, Patient Education, and Preventive Measures

Cognitive Level: Apply

37. 12–13 years old

Blueprint Task: Applying Basic Scientific Concepts

Cognitive Level: Recall

38. Chandelier sign

Chandelier sign is seen with cervical motion tenderness. This sign may be positive in conditions such as pelvic inflammatory disease, ectopic pregnancy, and appendicitis.

Blueprint Task: History Taking and Performing Physical Examination

Cognitive Level: Apply

39. Detection of premature rupture of membranes

Fern frond pattern of the vaginal secretions detects amniotic fluid and indicates the onset of labor. The fern test can also be used to detect ovulation and assist in fertility.

Blueprint Task: Using Diagnostic and Laboratory Studies

Cognitive Level: Apply

40. Full cervical dilation

Blueprint Task: Applying Basic Scientific Concepts

Cognitive Level: Recall

41. Developmental dysplasia of the hip (DDH)

The clinical vignette describes a frank breech presentation. Breech presentation increases the risk of DDH, commonly referred to as hip dysplasia. Additional risk factors include first-born, female gender, and positive family history.

Blueprint Task: Clinical Intervention

Cognitive Level: Analyze

42. What approach is used during a physical exam to assess fetal position in the abdomen during the later stages of pregnancy?

43. A 24-year-old woman has been trying to become pregnant for the past 10 months without success. She has been amenorrheic for the past 3 months. History is notable for weight gain and hirsutism. Previous labs demonstrated glucose intolerance, for which lifestyle modifications have been ineffective. Pelvic ultrasound shows polycystic ovaries. What pharmacologic therapy may improve fertility and decrease blood glucose?

44. What are the two high-risk HPV genotypes that cause the majority of high-risk cervical lesions and cervical cancer?

45. A 58-year-old woman with a history of chronic constipation and elevated body mass index presents with intermittent sensation of fullness in her vagina. Her occupation is associated with frequent heavy lifting. During Valsalva maneuver, there is protrusion of the anterior vaginal wall. What is the most likely diagnosis?

46. A 55-year-old woman who has not had a menstrual period for 3 years presents with vaginal bleeding. Pelvic exam reveals no vaginal ulceration or source of bleeding. What imaging study is recommended?

47. In healthy low-risk patients, what is the typical timing of an anatomical ultrasound to screen for fetal anomalies?

48. A 55-year-old woman presents with insomnia and vasomotor symptoms associated with menopause. She has an intact uterus and ovaries. What medication combination may be utilized to decrease her symptoms?

49. A 29-year-old woman describes occasional pelvic pain that occurs at the time of ovulation. What is this cyclic pain?

(See answers next page.)

42. Leopold maneuvers

Blueprint Task: History Taking and Performing Physical Examination
Cognitive Level: Recall

43. Metformin

The clinical vignette supports the diagnosis of polycystic ovarian syndrome. Androgen lowering medications can be utilized to treat hirsutism. Additional medications may be considered if spontaneous ovulation does not occur with metformin and are preferred in patients without glucose intolerance.
Blueprint Task: Pharmaceutical Therapeutics
Cognitive Level: Analyze

44. 16 and 18

Blueprint Task: Health Maintenance, Patient Education, and Preventive Measures
Cognitive Level: Recall

45. Cystocele

Increased abdominal pressure from repetitive lifting or straining with defecation raise the likelihood of cystocele development.
Blueprint Task: Formulating Most Likely Diagnosis
Cognitive Level: Apply

46. Transvaginal ultrasound

The clinical vignette supports the diagnosis of postmenopausal bleeding, which warrants additional work-up. The pelvic ultrasound will provide information regarding endometrial thickness and may be followed by an endometrial biopsy.
Blueprint Task: Using Diagnostic and Laboratory Studies
Cognitive Level: Apply

47. 18–20 weeks' gestation

Blueprint Task: Clinical Intervention
Cognitive Level: Recall

48. Estrogen and progesterone

In patients with intact uterus and ovaries experiencing distressing symptoms related to menopause, estrogen given without progesterone can lead to endometrial proliferation and increase the possibility of malignancy of the endometrium.
Blueprint Task: Pharmaceutical Therapeutics
Cognitive Level: Apply

49. Mittelschmerz

Blueprint Task: History Taking and Performing Physical Examination
Cognitive Level: Recall

50. A 48-year-old woman presents to the clinic with long-standing irregular heavy menstrual periods with cramping. On pelvic exam, the uterus is nontender; however, firm, mobile, and enlarged with nodularity. Laboratory evaluation reveals a negative pregnancy test and iron deficiency anemia. Ultrasound is used to confirm this condition. What is the most likely diagnosis?

51. A 23-year-old sexually active woman presents with malodorous, gray vaginal discharge. Testing for sexually transmitted infection (STI) is negative; however, wet mount reveals epithelial cells covered with bacteria. What type of cells are associated with the presumptive diagnosis?

52. During the first prenatal visit, a 23-year-old woman is determined to be negative for the Rh (D) antigen without anti-D alloimmunization. What medical intervention should be provided at 28 weeks' gestation to prevent complications related to Rh incompatibility?

53. A 60-year-old woman presents to the clinic with vaginal dryness and soreness during intercourse which has progressively worsened over the last 5 years. On physical exam, the vaginal mucosa is pale with decreased rugae; no lesions are noted. What is the presumptive diagnosis?

54. What intramuscular medication may be utilized to decrease the risk of preterm, premature rupture of the membranes in a patient with a history of preterm deliveries?

55. A 32-year-old woman presents to the clinic with postcoital vaginal bleeding, pelvic fullness, and occasional dysuria. Her last Papanicolaou test was 10 years ago and normal. What finding on physical exam would necessitate a referral for biopsy?

56. What is the most common cause of postpartum hemorrhage?

57. A 30-year-old woman with a history of hypertension, tobacco, and cocaine use presents to the emergency department at 34 weeks' gestation. She is experiencing uterine contractions and bright red vaginal bleeding with pelvic and abdominal pain. There is no history of trauma. What is the presumptive diagnosis?

(See answers next page.)

50. Uterine leiomyoma

Uterine leiomyoma, also called fibroid tumor, is the most common benign cause of uterine tumor. While irregular bleeding and pain are common manifestations, patients with leiomyomas may be asymptomatic.

Blueprint Task: *Formulating Most Likely Diagnosis*
Cognitive Level: *Analyze*

51. Clue cells

The clinical vignette supports the diagnosis of bacterial vaginosis (BV). Sexual activity is a risk factor for developing BV, although the infection is not an STI.

Blueprint Task: *Using Diagnostic and Laboratory Studies*
Cognitive Level: *Analyze*

52. Rh immunoglobulin (RhIg)

Blueprint Task: *Clinical Intervention*
Cognitive Level: *Recall*

53. Genitourinary syndrome of menopause

Vaginal atrophy is due to chronic estrogen deficiency. Topical estrogen therapy is recommended unless contraindicated.

Blueprint Task: *Formulating Most Likely Diagnosis*
Cognitive Level: *Apply*

54. 17-α hydroxyprogesterone caproate

Blueprint Task: *Pharmaceutical Therapeutics*
Cognitive Level: *Recall*

55. Cervical lesion

The historical features within the clinical vignette and an associated cervical lesion would be concerning for cancer. Referral for biopsy is indicated.

Blueprint Task: *History Taking and Performing Physical Examination*
Cognitive Level: *Analyze*

56. Uterine atony

Blueprint Task: *Applying Basic Scientific Concepts*
Cognitive Level: *Recall*

57. Placental abruption

The clinical vignette outlines risk factors for placental abruption, such as tobacco, cocaine use, and history of hypertension. Other risk factors include a bleeding disorder or a previous abruption.

Blueprint Task: *Formulating Most Likely Diagnosis*
Cognitive Level: *Apply*

58. What medication is recommended to be given intravenously to a pregnant patient in active labor with severe genital herpes simplex infection?

59. A 24-year-old woman presents with right-sided vaginal pain and dyspareunia for a week. Physical exam reveals a warm, erythematous, tender, and fluctuant mass measuring 3 cm in diameter, lateral to the vaginal opening. What is the most likely diagnosis?

60. A 25-year-old woman presents with concerns of infertility. She describes long-standing pelvic pain, dysmenorrhea, and dyspareunia. Previous evaluation of her symptoms revealed abnormal deposition of endometrial tissue outside of the uterus. What is the most likely diagnosis based on this historical presentation?

61. What is the recommended clinical intervention for a pregnant patient with cervical insufficiency?

62. At how many weeks' gestation are fetal heart sounds typically first detectable by doppler?

63. A 53-year-old woman presents to the clinic with progressive hot flashes, irritability, night sweats, and decreased libido. Her last menstrual period was over 2 years ago. What is the most likely diagnosis?

64. A 30-year-old woman is 29 weeks' gestation and in preterm labor. What first-line class of medication may be administered to the mother to increase fetal lung maturity?

65. A 29-year-old woman with a history of ovarian cysts presents to the emergency department with acute onset of severe, left-side lower abdominal pain. Physical exam reveals guarding over the left lower abdomen along with left-sided adnexal tenderness on bimanual exam. Serum beta-hCG is negative. Doppler ultrasound shows decreased arterial flow to the left adnexa. What is the presumptive diagnosis?

66. How many weeks gestation would you expect the fundal height to be at the level of the umbilicus in a normal singleton pregnancy?

(See answers next page.)

58. Acyclovir
Blueprint Task: Pharmaceutical Therapeutics
Cognitive Level: Recall

59. Bartholin gland abscess
Additional symptoms of a Bartholin gland abscess may include pain with walking or sitting and spontaneous drainage. Bartholin gland cysts are typically asymptomatic unless sizable.
Blueprint Task: Formulating Most Likely Diagnosis
Cognitive Level: Apply

60. Endometriosis
Blueprint Task: History Taking and Performing Physical Examination
Cognitive Level: Recall

61. Cervical cerclage
A cerclage uses suture to reinforce the cervix and decrease the risk of premature labor.
Blueprint Task: Clinical Intervention
Cognitive Level: Apply

62. 10–12 weeks
Blueprint Task: History Taking and Performing Physical Examination
Cognitive Level: Recall

63. Menopause
Vasomotor symptoms are experienced by a majority of women going through menopause and frequently last 5 years or more.
Blueprint Task: Formulating Most Likely Diagnosis
Cognitive Level: Apply

64. Corticosteroid
Blueprint Task: Pharmaceutical Therapeutics
Cognitive Level: Recall

65. Ovarian torsion
Ovarian torsion is a medical emergency. A positive doppler study is highly predictive, but a negative study does not rule out the diagnosis. Gynecology should be involved if ovarian torsion is suspected clinically.
Blueprint Task: Formulating Most Likely Diagnosis
Cognitive Level: Apply

66. 20 weeks
Blueprint Task: History Taking and Performing Physical Examination
Cognitive Level: Recall

Professional Practice

1. What three medical interventions are subject to conscientious objection for a provider?

2. What terminology does the American Academy of Physician Assistants (AAPA) use to describe collaborative practice for PAs that highlights the desire to continue to work closely in teams with physicians, while eliminating the requirements of having a supervising physician to allow the PA to practice?

3. What organization performs interval site visits of healthcare organizations and uses tracer methodology to assess quality and performance improvement measures to ensure the delivery of safe and effective patient care?

4. What term describes the systematic contrast in medical care received based on cultural or socioeconomic backgrounds and may compromise patient safety and increase the risk of poor patient outcomes?

5. A 56-year-old woman with metastatic breast cancer to the liver and lungs has been advised that her illness is terminal and unlikely to improve. Given her prognosis, what document directs medical care related to withholding or removing life-preserving therapy?

6. Clinicians are legally required to notify state or local agencies, such as child protective services, if abuse or neglect is suspected. What term defines this role?

7. A 19-year-old woman presents to the emergency department with signs and symptoms consistent with uncomplicated cystitis. During the exam, she discloses to the clinician that she has been an unwilling participant in a sex trafficking operation. What organization can the clinician contact for instruction on risk assessment, management, and available resources?

8. A patient presents to the cardiac catheterization lab for a non-emergent cardiac angiography. In the event of respiratory or cardiac arrest, what pre-procedural order outlines direction regarding initiation or discontinuation of life-sustaining treatment?

9. What organ system encompasses the largest amount of content in the PANCE and PANRE?

10. A clinician working in the emergency department becomes aware of a colleague's repeated breach of patient confidentiality. The clinician is not sure if this breach was intentional or unintentional. Given HIPAA guidelines, after the discovery of the breach, who should the clinician promptly notify to most effectively handle the situation?

(See answers next page.) **243**

1. Abortion, contraception, and sterilization

Conscientious objection is a protected right of a clinician to morally object to a particular intervention based on personal beliefs.

Cognitive Level: Apply

2. Optimal team practice

Cognitive Level: Recall

3. Joint Commission on Accreditation of Healthcare Organizations (JCAHO)

Cognitive Level: Recall

4. Healthcare disparities

Cognitive Level: Recall

5. Living will

This advanced directive would supersede a Medical Power of Attorney once a patient becomes incapacitated.

Cognitive Level: Apply

6. Mandated reporter

Cognitive Level: Recall

7. National Human Trafficking Resource Center

Cognitive Level: Recall

8. Do not resuscitate orders (DNR Orders)

Cognitive Level: Recall

9. Cardiovascular

Cognitive Level: Recall

10. Hospital legal counsel

Clinics often name a privacy officer to fulfill this role. A breach includes unlawful access, utilization, or the release of protected health information.

Cognitive Level: Apply

11. What law was enacted in 1985 that outlines the requirements for hospital emergency departments to perform a medical screening exam and evaluate for emergent medical conditions in all patients regardless of insurance coverage or legal status?

12. Prior to performing a medical procedure, the clinician must be certain of what two elements predicating informed consent on the part of the patient?

13. A practitioner discovers he will not be covered by his current malpractice plan once he leaves the practice. What type of policy would provide extended coverage?

14. In the emergency department, a patient refuses the recommended treatment and voices the desire to leave without receiving medical care. Why is it important that the clinician have the patient sign a discharge against-medical-advice form?

15. Patients may experience harm during an inpatient admission due to pharmaceutical side effects or medication errors. What term describes this harmful event?

16. Disaster preparedness is an essential aspect of hospital administration. Once a disaster has been identified, what is the predetermined area within the hospital that will serve as a central command and control facility and maintain communication with the emergency department, triage, and external authorities?

17. A 56-year-old man is hospitalized with COVID-19. Prior to entering the room to initiate patient care, what type of specialized equipment should be worn by the provider to reduce the risk of exposure?

18. During a disaster, hospitals often must care for high volumes of patients. What is the term defined by an emergency department's ability to provide care to a higher quantity of patients than is routine for the organization?

19. An outbreak of measles is identified in a community. A 12-year-old boy with an unknown vaccination history is found to have had a measles exposure. What is the best course of action to protect the patient?

20. The Vessel Sanitation Program, established by the CDC, has led to a decrease in the spread of gastrointestinal illnesses in travelers aboard cruise ships. What is the most common viral pathogen causing gastroenteritis in these individuals?

21. A healthy 34-year-old man is traveling to Africa for the first time. His immunizations are current. What additional live vaccine is recommended prior to travel?

22. CPT provides a consistent method to report medical, surgical, diagnostic services, and procedures. What does this billing and coding acronym stand for?

(*See answers next page.*)

11. Emergency Medical Treatment and Active Labor Act (EMTALA)
Cognitive Level: Recall

12. Decision-making capacity and free choice
Cognitive Level: Recall

13. Tail coverage
Tail (also referred to as Extended Reporting Period) may be purchased as limited or indefinite coverage based on the duration of continued coverage beyond the termination date of the claims-made policy. A claims-made policy is triggered by the date the claim was made and not based on when the incident occurred.
Cognitive Level: Apply

14. Provides documentation of medical treatment refusal
Cognitive Level: Recall

15. Adverse drug event (ADE)
Cognitive Level: Recall

16. Emergency operations center
Cognitive Level: Recall

17. Personal protective equipment (PPE)
PPE may include gloves, face mask, gown, or additional considerations depending on the potential exposure.
Cognitive Level: Apply

18. Surge capacity
Cognitive Level: Recall

19. Immunization
Immunization against measles is recommended as soon as possible post-exposure. Proactive measures are recommended to minimize the spread of the highly contagious virus.
Cognitive Level: Apply

20. Norovirus
Cognitive Level: Recall

21. Yellow fever
Portions of Africa and South America are endemic for Yellow fever transmission. Clinicians are encouraged to check the CDC website for travel medicine risk information.
Cognitive Level: Apply

22. Current Procedural Terminology (CPT)
Cognitive Level: Recall

23. A 52-year-old man presents to the emergency department with an acute GI bleed, hypotension, and significant anemia. As a Jehovah's Witness, what primary therapeutic treatment may be declined by the patient?

24. What is the study and analysis of the distribution and determinants of infectious and noninfectious disease that focuses on surveillance, acquisition, transmission, management, and prevention?

25. Vertical transmission of a pathogen may occur during gestation across the placenta, during delivery, and through what other mechanism?

26. A child newly diagnosed with deafness is receiving coordinated care by her primary care provider and specialists in the fields of audiology, speech-language pathology, and otolaryngology. They routinely meet to discuss and create care plans for delivering services. What term describes this type of healthcare team collaboration?

27. Along with insect repellents, bed nets, and other measures to reduce frequency of mosquito bites, what other malaria prevention strategy should be discussed with patients prior to travel to endemic areas?

28. What syndrome, defined by emotional exhaustion, depersonalization, and low sense of personal accomplishment, has been associated with poor job performance?

29. What two main components focus on palliative end-of-life care?

30. An experienced provider discovers that he made a medical error that resulted in a poor patient outcome. What primary action is ethically appropriate and reestablishes informed consent in the continuation of care?

31. What is the most common factor influencing the decision-making process of a patient seeking malpractice litigation against a provider?

32. Postexposure prophylaxis after a high-risk needle stick is available for what two viral infections?

33. A clinician is gowned and gloved for surgery. What areas of the clinician's body are considered sterile following proper gowning and gloving?

34. A local company offers a healthcare provider a financial incentive every time she orders a particular diagnostic test. The business agreement is stimulating referrals for this test even when it may not be necessary for optimal patient care. What ethical scenario does this represent?

35. A family just learned that their loved one is dying. Based on federal regulations in the United States, who is recommended to initiate the conversation with the family to obtain consent for organ donation?

(See answers next page.)

23. Blood transfusion

The clinician should thoughtfully discuss a patient's cultural and religious beliefs without assumption or judgment. Preferably, these conversations are recommended prior to the development of a medical need.

Cognitive Level: Apply

24. Epidemiology

Cognitive Level: Recall

25. Breastfeeding

Cognitive Level: Recall

26. Interprofessional

Cognitive Level: Recall

27. Chemoprophylaxis

Malaria chemoprophylaxis is not completely protective. Therapeutic recommendations vary based on geographic locations and local drug sensitivities.

Cognitive Level: Apply

28. Burnout

Cognitive Level: Recall

29. Symptom control and quality of life

Cognitive Level: Recall

30. Disclosure of the medical error

Disclosure reinforces trust and integrity, which can strengthen the patient–provider relationship. Informed consent cannot be upheld if there are undisclosed errors.

Cognitive Level: Apply

31. The patient perceives a poor patient–provider relationship

Cognitive Level: Recall

32. Hepatitis B and HIV

Cognitive Level: Recall

33. Gloved hands to the shoulder and front of gown to the waist

Cognitive Level: Recall

34. Conflict of interest

Conflict of interest occurs when a provider's interest supersedes the interest of a patient.

Cognitive Level: Apply

35. Organ Procurement Organization (OPO)

Cognitive Level: Recall

36. A clinician becomes increasingly concerned about the safety of a colleague and the safety of her patients. The clinician has smelled alcohol on her breath daily and has noted her to be more irritable, moody, and frequently absent from work. How should the clinician respond to this situation?

37. What area of medicine focuses on target therapies to maximize benefits and minimize side effects, based on personalized factors such as genetics and biomarkers?

38. How many Category 1 CME credits are required for PAs to recertify per 2-year cycle based on the National Commission on Certification of Physician Assistants (NCCPA) requirements?

39. A clinician has an exceptionally busy day in the emergency department. He recognizes 4 days after a shift that he forgot to document a patient visit in the electronic health record (EHR). How should the clinician proceed with documentation of the visit?

40. What entity is the single, largest payer for healthcare in the United States?

41. The evaluation and management (E/M) level of CPT coding is determined by the patient's history, physical exam, and medical decision-making. A fourth component, time, may also be included in the E/M level for counseling and coordination of care when the time spent consumes at least what percentage of the total visit time?

42. A language barrier is impacting communication during a non-emergent office visit. A 9-year-old grandchild of the patient offers to assist with communication. How should the clinician respond to this offer?

43. A terminally ill patient requests that her clinician prescribe a lethal dose of medication due to her severity of physical and emotional suffering. What term describes this legally sanctioned process?

44. What committee provides approval of clinical research design and methods to ensure ethical regulations are upheld and to protect human subjects?

45. The Triple Aim was transformed into the Quadruple Aim by adding what goal?

46. What is the designated group within the hospital that directs and problem solves ethical healthcare dilemmas such as confidentiality, informed consent, and end-of-life issues?

47. How can physician assistants bill under a collaborating physician's Provider Identification Number (PIN) when the physician is not present for the encounter?

48. A patient is hospitalized with *Clostridioides difficile* colitis and has orders for strict contact precautions. Upon leaving the patient's room, what is the recommended approach to prevent spread by the provider?

(See answers next page.)

36. Report concerns about clinician impairment

The duty to report is guided by a medical board's focus on protecting the public. The clinician should report to the appropriate entity based on the practice setting.

Cognitive Level: Apply

37. Precision medicine

Cognitive Level: Recall

38. 50

Cognitive Level: Recall

39. Late entry documentation

The late entry is to include documentation of the time/date and a brief rationale for delay.

Cognitive Level: Apply

40. Medicare

Cognitive Level: Recall

41. 50%

Cognitive Level: Recall

42. Decline and obtain a professional interpreter

Young children should not be used as interpreters, except in life-threatening emergencies.

Cognitive Level: Apply

43. Physician-assisted death

Cognitive Level: Recall

44. Institutional review board (IRB)

Cognitive Level: Recall

45. Attain joy at work

The other goals of the Quadruple Aim include improving the health of populations, enhancing the patient experience, and reducing healthcare costs.

Cognitive Level: Apply

46. Ethics committee

Cognitive Level: Recall

47. Incident-to billing

Cognitive Level: Recall

48. Wash hands

Washing hands with soap and water is recommended. Alcohol-based antiseptics may not effectively eliminate certain pathogens, such as *C. difficile*.

Cognitive Level: Apply

Index

abdominal aortic aneurysm (AAA), 23, 28, 84
acanthosis nigricans, 52
acetazolamide, 66
acoustic neuromas, 74
acromegaly, 58
acromioclavicular (AC) joint injury, 155
acute arterial occlusion, 12
acute bronchitis, 196
acute coronary syndrome (ACS), 11
acute flaccid paralysis, 172
acute hepatitis B infection, 96
acute kidney injury (AKI), 220
acute lymphoblastic leukemia (ALL), 116
acute mesenteric ischemia, 96
acute myeloid leukemia (AML), 114
acute prostatitis, 104
acute respiratory distress syndrome (ARDS), 206
acute rheumatic fever (ARF), 28, 128
acute simple cystitis, 112
acute tubular necrosis, 222
acyclovir, 242
adenomas, 88
adrenal gland, 60
adverse drug event (ADE), 246
agoraphobia, 180
allen test, 14
allergic conjunctivitis, 76
allopurinol, 156
alpha-adrenergic receptor antagonists, 110
alpha-fetoprotein (AFP), 90, 102
5-alpha-reductase inhibitors, 102
ambulatory devices, 10
amenorrhea, 178
American Academy of Pediatrics (AAP), 161, 166
American Academy of Physician Assistants (AAPA), 243
amoxicillin-clavulanate, 62
amyloidosis, 2
anal squamous cell carcinoma, 84
anesthetics, 86
angioedema, 78
angiotensin-converting enzyme (ACE), 1, 9, 25, 28, 214, 216, 220

angiotensin-converting enzyme inhibitors (ACE-I), 53
angiotensin receptor blocker (ARB), 26, 53, 214, 216, 220
anisocytosis, 115
ankle-brachial index (ABI), 20
anorexia nervosa, 177
anterior interosseus nerve (AIN), 142
anthelmintic, 134
antibiotic prophylaxis, 10
antibiotics
    Clostridioides diffic, 89
    cystitis, 105
    dermatologic system, 38
    empiric antibiotic therapy, 70, 72, 78, 82, 84, 120, 164, 186, 229
    gastrointestinal system/nutrition, 88
    genitourinary system, 101
    infectious diseases, 126
    musculoskeletal system, 141
    neurologic system, 159
    oral, 130
    otic, 76
    pulmonary system, 195
    topical, 71, 132
anticoagulation, 120
antidiuretic hormone (ADH), 46, 58
antihistamine, 76
anti-mitochondrial antibody, 92
anti-müllerian hormone (AMH), 228
antineutrophil cytoplasmic antibodies (ANCA), 149
antiphospholipid syndrome, 118
antipsychotics, 176
anti-streptolysin (ASO), 27
aortic regurgitation (AR), 26
aortic root dilation, 2
aortic stenosis, 14
aortic valve stenosis, 22
arrhythmia, 9, 11, 15, 17, 20, 55, 223, 224
asbestosis, 208
ascending cholangitis, 80
ascites, 90

ascorbic acid, 118
aspirin, 6, 116
asymmetric flaccid paralysis, 172
atelectasis, 204
atherosclerotic cardiovascular disease
    (ASCVD), 50
atlantoaxial instability (AAI), 166
atorvastatin, 22
atrial fibrillation, 56
atrioventricular block, 4
atropine, 22
attention deficit hyperactivity disorder
    (ADHD), 168, 176, 178, 184
atypical lymphocytes, 62
audiometry, 74
auditory hallucinations, 179
autism spectrum disorder (ASD), 177, 188
azithromycin, 126

bacitracin, 68
bacterial vaginosis (BV), 240
barium enema, 88
"barking seal," 69
Barlow test, 140
Barrett esophagus, 96
bartholin gland abscess, 242
basal cell carcinoma (BCC), 38
Bell's palsy, 163
benzodiazepine, 174, 186
beriberi, 79
beta-blockers, 1, 2, 6, 10, 12, 28, 184
beta subunit of the human chorionic
    gonadotropin (beta-hCG), 102
beta-thalassemia, 124
bigeminy, 24
bile acid binding resins, 6
bismuth subsalicylate, 94
bisphosphonates, 144, 156
bladder rupture, 110
blurred vision, 102
bracing, 156
bronchiectasis, 212
bronchiolitis, 195
bruit, 22
bupropion, 194
bursal aspiration, 148

calcium pyrophosphate crystal (CPPD)
    deposition disease, 150
Campylobacter jejuni, 136
cardiac auscultation, 3

cardiogenic shock, 5, 14
cardiovascular system
    aorta, coarctation of the, 18
    beta-blockers, 1, 2, 6, 10, 12, 28
    catheter ablation, 18
    family history, 24
    graft rejection, 26
    left, lower sternal border, 28
    NSAIDs, 6
    ST-segment elevation, 18, 20, 24
    TEE, 16
    ultrasound, 6
    widened mediastinum, 26
cauda equina syndrome, 156
ceftriaxone, 126
celiac disease, 100
central retinal artery occlusion (CRAO), 76
central retinal vascular occlusion (CRVO), 72
cephalosporin, 158
cerebrospinal fluid (CSF), 161
chemical urethritis, 110
chemoprophylaxis, 248
chest discomfort, 5
chest radiograph, 15
Cheyne Stokes breathing, 204
Chlamydia trachomatis, 130
chordee, 108
chronic candidal vulvovaginitis, 47
chronic kidney disease (CKD), 213
chronic lymphocytic leukemia (CLL), 120
chronic myeloid leukemia (CML), 117
chronic obstructive lung disease (COPD), 203
chronic obstructive pulmonary disease
    (COPD), 192, 193, 211
chronic venous insufficiency, 10
ciprofloxacin, 76
cirrhosis, 80, 89, 98
Clostridioides difficile, 89
clue cells, 240
cognitive behavioral psychotherapy, 180
colchicine, 6
colon cancer, 100
colovesical fistula, 110
community-acquired pneumonia (CAP), 197
compartment syndrome, 144
complete blood count (CBC), 117, 178
complex regional pain syndrome (CRPS), 170
compression stockings, 8
conduct disorder (CD), 178
conductive hearing loss, 62
congenital hypothyroidism, 45, 46

congestive heart failure (CHF), 3, 16, 193
conjunctival injection, 162
contact lens, 106
continuous positive airway pressure
    (CPAP), 196
copper intrauterine device (IUD), 236
corneal ulcer, 78
coronavirus disease 2019 (COVID-19), 210
cor pulmonale, 4
corrigan pulse, 25, 26
corticosteroid injection, 152
corticosteroids, 70, 78, 86, 122, 152, 200
costovertebral angle (CVA) tenderness, 214
Cosyntropin (ACTH) stimulation test, 48
cranial nerve III, 72
cranial nerves (CN), 169
cremasteric reflex, 106
CREST syndrome, 152
cretinism, 46
Crohn disease, 87, 98
CT scan
    endocrine system, 51
    gastrointestinal system/nutrition, 86
current procedural terminology (CPT), 246
Cushing's syndrome, 55, 60
cutaneous larva migrans (CLM), 128
cyanosis, 202
cystic fibrosis (CF), 212
cystoscopy, 104
cytomegalovirus (CMV), 128

daily Amsler grid checks, 64
dal anti-platelet therapy (DAPT), 11, 12
debridement, 72
deep vein thrombosis (DVT), 9, 12, 13
dehydroepiandrosterone (DHEA), 59
dementia with Lewy body (DLB), 162
dental erosion, 180
depigmentation, 29
de Quervain's tenosynovitis, 150
dermatitis herpetiformis, 84
dermatologic system
    antibiotics, 38
    antifungal, 32
    atypical target lesion, 34
    biopsy, 40
    bright appearing mass, 36
    CBC, 34
    histology, 30
    imaging modalities, 32
    incision and drainage, 32

keratinization, 42
lice and nits, 42
lipid panel, 34
liver test, 34
mark the borders, 36
pregnancy test, 34
pressure reducing devices, 34
SJS, 34
smoking cessation, 32
SPF, 33
superficial partial thickness, 42
ultraviolet (UV), 34
umbilicated dome-shaped papule, 36
weight management, 32
dermatomyositis, 144
desmopressin, 44, 118
developmental dysplasia of the hip
    (DDH), 236
dexamethasone, 168
dexamethasone suppression test, 56
dextrocardia, 24
diabetes insipidus, 46
diabetes mellitus, 32, 48
diabetic ketoacidosis (DKA), 54, 57
diabetic neuropathy, 185
diabetic retinopathy, 60
diastolic murmur, 23
Dietary Approaches to Stop Hypertension
    (DASH) diet, 22
diphtheria, 130
direct immunofluorescence microscopy, 30
disease-modifying antirheumatic drugs
    (DMARDs), 154
distal interphalangeal (DIP), 142
disulfiram, 180
diuretics, 8, 84
do not resuscitate orders (DNR Orders), 244
dorsalis pedis, 12
doxycycline, 126, 138
dual-energy x-ray absorptiometry (DXA),
    47, 152
duodenal ulcer, 90
dysdiadochokinesia, 160
dysphagia, 94
dysthymia, 184

echocardiogram, 4
ecthyma, 34
ectopic pregnancy, 230
ectropion, 72
ejection fraction, 7

elastic graduated compression stockings, 16
electrical alternans, 8
electrocardiogram (ECG), 1, 2, 3, 7, 9–11, 14,
    15, 17, 19, 21, 23, 185, 215
electroconvulsive therapy (ECT), 190
electroencephalography (EEG), 170
elongated filiform papillae, 76
Emergency Medical Treatment and Active
    Labor Act (EMTALA), 246
emphysema, 200
empiric antibiotic therapy, 70, 72, 78, 82, 94,
    120, 164, 186, 229
empiric systemic antibiotic therapy, 64
endocrine system
    ADH, 46
    antiemetics, 56
    CT scan, 51
    FNA biopsy, 44
    HbA1C, 52
    HHS, 44
    IV fluids, 58
    nonproliferative, 58
    overweight, 50
    primary hyperparathyroidism, 44
    promotility agents, 56
    PTH, 50
    regular exercise, 52
    rotation of injection sites, 54
    "socking and glove," 50
    vitamin D, 44
    weight-bearing, 48
enemas, 98
eosinophils, 118
epididymitis, 112
epiglottis, 71
epinephrine, 212
Epley maneuver, 68
Epstein- Barr virus, 62
erysipelas, 38
erythema infectiosum, 40
erythema migrans, 138
erythematous facial rash, 37
erythrocyte sedimentation rate (ESR), 27
erythromycin ointment, 68
erythropoiesis-stimulating agents, 214
Escherichia coli, 102
esophageal candidiasis, 138
esophageal manometry, 96
esophagogastroduodenoscopy (EGD), 81, 92,
    93, 97, 99

estrogen cream, 106
evaluation and management (E/M), 249
extended focused assessment with
    sonography for trauma (eFAST), 12
extracorporeal shock wave lithotripsy, 112
extraocular movements (EOMs), 169

factitious disorder, 188
Felty syndrome, 120
ferritin, 120
fever, 92
fibromyalgia, 185
fidaxomicin, 90
fine-needle aspiration (FNA) biopsy, 44
flank mass, 218
flank pain, 218
fluconazole, 132
fluid resuscitation, 5
fluorescein stain, 72
fluoroquinolones, 76, 110, 216
folate, 88
folic acid, 170
food-borne botulism, 132
fragile X syndrome (FXS), 164
fungal scalp dermatitis, 37
furosemide, 38
furuncle, 34

galactorrhea, 234
gallbladder cancer, 80
gallbladder polyps, 79
gastric emptying scan, 80
gastrin, 94
gastroenteropancreatic neuroendocrine
    tumors (GEP-NET), 51
gastrointestinal system/nutrition
    antibiotic use, 88
    antifungal, 98
    atopy, 82
    CT scan, 86
    dietary phenylalanine restriction, 92
    empiric antibiotic, 82, 94
    excision, 84
    exercise, 92
    hospitalization, 88
    NSAIDs, 80
    right upper quadrant (RUQ), 95
    sigmoid volvulus, 82
    surgical pyloromyotomy, 88
    therapeutic phlebotomy, 88

trichobezoar, removal of, 90
ultrasonography, 90
ultrasound, 98
unconjugated hyperbilirubinemia, 90
gastrointestinal toxicity, 142
generalized anxiety disorder (GAD), 186
genitourinary syndrome, 240
genitourinary system
    antifungal, 108
    dorsal, 106
    imaging studies, 104
    orchiopexy, 108
    post-void residual volume, 106
    transrectal ultrasound-guided biopsy, 108
gestational diabetes mellitus (GDM), 229
giant cell arteritis, 18
gigantism, 46
Gilbert syndrome, 90
Global Initiative for Chronic Obstructive
    Lung Disease (GOLD), 203
glucocorticoids, 148, 198
glucose, 46
glucose tolerance test, 230
gonioscopy, 64
Goodpasture syndrome, 222
granulomatosis with polyangiitis (GPA), 214
Graves' orbitopathy, 56
Guillain-Barré syndrome, 171

Haemophilus influenzae B, 72
Haemophilus influenzae type b (Hib)
    vaccine, 210
hamartoma, 206
hand, foot and mouth disease (HFMD), 132
Hashimoto's thyroiditis, 47, 58
Hawkins impingement test, 152
Helicobacter pylori, 82
hematologic system
    daily oral iron replacement, 118
    dehydration, 114
    empiric antibiotics, 120
    factor VIII deficiency, 114
    fever, 122
    gastric biopsy, 116
    heavy menses, 114
    hemoglobin, 114
    hypercoagulability, 118
    pallor, 120
    red blood cell size, 116
    stasis, 118
    vessel wall injury, 118

hematopoietic stem cell transplant, 124
hematuria, 218
hemolytic uremic syndrome, 84
hemorrhagic nontender lesions, 3
heparin, 114, 120
heparin-induced thrombocytopenia (HIT), 24
hepatitis A virus (HAV) infection, 88
hepatitis B virus, 150
hepatojugular reflux, 20
hereditary spherocytosis, 116
herpes simplex keratitis, 62
herpes simplex virus, 130
high-sensitivity troponin testing, 8
hordeolum, 68
Horner syndrome, 212
human papillomavirus (HPV), 108
Huntington's disease, 172
hydrocele, 110
hydroxychloroquine, 140
hyperactivity-impulsivity, 183
hyperaldosteronism, 48
hyperbaric oxygen therapy, 168, 206
hyperkalemia, 2
hyperkyphosis, 154
hyperosmolar hyperglycemic state (HHS), 44
hyperphosphatemia, 56, 216
hypertensive emergency, 28
hyperthyroidism, 58
hypertrophic cardiomyopathy, 8
hypoactive sexual desire disorder (HSSD), 110
hypocalcemia, 46
hypogonadotropic hypogonadism, 54
hyponatremia, 58
hypopigmentation, 29
hypospadias, 102
hypotension, 92

idiopathic thrombocytopenic purpura
    (ITP), 122
ileus, 90
immune thrombocytopenia (ITP), 116, 121
immunoglobulin A (IgA) vasculitis, 122
implantable cardioverter defibrillator (ICD), 7
implanted intrathecal pump (ITP), 169
inactivated poliovirus (IPV), 133
indomethacin, 8
infectious diseases
    anterior nares, 134
    beta-hemolytic *Streptococci*, 132
    blood culture, 136
    chancre, 136

infectious diseases (*continued*)
   chemoprophylaxis, 130
   coccidioidomycosis, 138
   environmental, 132
   erythematous macular, 138
   ethambutol, 138
   fluid resuscitation, 126
   histoplasmosis, 134
   HIV1/HIV2 combination antigen/antibody
     immunoassay, 130
   IgM, 128
   incision and drainage, 130
   intranasal, 136
   isoniazid, 138
   pyrazinamide, 138
   rifampin, 138
   target lesions, 134
   TDap, 126
   topical antibiotic, 132
   T. vaginalis, 130
inferior rectus, 64
inflammatory bowel disease (IBD), 83
influenza vaccine, 132
inguinal hernia, 104
inhaled corticosteroids (ICS), 196
institutional review board (IRB), 250
insulin-like growth factor (IGF-1), 57
intercostal space, 4
interferon-gamma release assay (IGRA), 134
intermittent claudication, 28
international normalized ratio (INR), 54
intracranial bleeding, 2
intracranial pressure (ICP), 161
intranasal corticosteroid, 64, 66
intraocular pressure (IOP), 68
intravenous immune globulin (IVIG), 172
intravenous (IV) fluid replacement, 7
intussusception, 92
iron deficiency, 188
iron-deficiency anemia, 116
irritable bowel syndrome (IBS), 96
ischemic chest pain, 13
ischemic heart disease, 4
isotretinoin, 33, 184

janeway lesions, 4
Janus Kinase 2 gene (JAK2), 121
Jefferson fracture, 142
jerk nystagmus, 64
Joint Commission on Accreditation of
   Healthcare Organizations (JCAHO), 244
jugular venous distension (JVD), 11

Kayser-Fleischer ring, 68
Kegel, 102
keratinization, 42
kerion, 38
Kiesselbach's plexus, 66
Klebsiella pneumoniae, 197
Klinefelter syndrome, 50
Kocher criteria, 154
Koebner phenomenon, 32
Koplik spots, 74

Lachman test, 144
lacrimation, 162
lactate dehydrogenase (LDH), 102
lactose intolerance, 86
lactulose, 96
left ventricular apical ballooning, 2
Legg-Calve-Perthes disease, 146
legionella, 196
Leiden mutation, 122
leukocytosis, 148
leukoplakia, 62
levine sign, 14
lichen planus, 31
light therapy, 182
lipohypertrophy, 54
lithium carbonate, 188
live attenuated influenza vaccine (LAIV), 207
long-acting insulin, 58
loop diuretics, 14
lower-extremity venous doppler
   ultrasound, 12
lupus nephritis, 224
lymphangitis, 30
lymphocytosis, 134

macrocytic anemia, 81
macrolides, 194
macular degeneration, 63
malar (butterfly) rash, 40
malignant melanoma, 29
Mallory-Weiss tear, 100
mannitol, 162
Marcus Gunn pupil, 164
marijuana, 182
measles, 74
meclizine, 76
medial ankle, 16
melasma, 230
Ménière's disease, 76
meningioma, 172
meniscus, 142

menstrual cycle, 212
metabolic acidosis, 194
metabolic syndrome, 28
metamorphopsia, 64
metastatic gastric adenocarcinoma, 86
metformin, 50, 238
methacholine, 194
methicillin-resistant *Staphylococcus aureus* (MRSA), 133
methimazole, 46
methotrexate, 232
methylprednisolone, 160
metoclopramide, 82
microcephaly, 136
minimal change disease (MCD), 216
Mini-Mental State Exam (MMSE), 173
minoxidil, 36
mitral stenosis, 9
mitral valve prolapse (MVP), 4
mitral valve stenosis, 24
Mittelschmerz, 238
Modified Checklist for Autism in Toddlers (M-CHAT), 161
molluscum contagiosum, 35
Monteggia fracture dislocation, 148
morbilliform rash, 126
multiple endocrine neoplasia (MEN) 1, 52
multiple sclerosis (MS), 161
mumps, 106, 136
mupirocin, 134
Murphy's sign, 96
muscle diseases, 22
muscle-strengthening activities, 25
musculoskeletal system
    A1 pulley, 144
    anti-CCP antibodies, 142
    axillary, 140
    breast, 150
    calcium channel blockers, 150
    discoloration, 158
    full extension, 156
    HLA-B27, 144
    internal rotation, 150
    L4-L5, 146
    laboratory studies, 148
    low back pain, 144
    lung, 150
    MR arthrogram, 140
    NSAIDs, 146
    "OK" sign, 142
    pain, 146
    patella, 148
    prostate, 150
    radial head reduction, 146
    sail sign, 146
    segmental fractures, 154
    urate crystals, 142
myocardial infarction (MI), 6, 19
myocarditis, 23
myositis, 22
myxoma, 18

Naegele's rule, 234
naloxone, 184
nasal polyps, 72
nasogastric (NG) tube, 100
National Commission on Certification of Physician Assistants (NCCPA), 249
National Human Trafficking Resource Center, 244
nebulized racemic epinephrine, 70
neovascularization, 54
neuraminidase inhibitors, 204
neurocognitive impairment, 46
neuroendocrine tumor, 5
neurofibromatosis type 2 (NF2), 73
neuroleptic malignant syndrome (NMS), 176
neurologic system
    absence seizures, 172
    advancing age, 174
    anti-convulsant, 174
    areflexia, 174
    automatisms, 168
    baclofen withdrawal, 170
    bacterial brain abscess, 160
    Brudzinski sign, 172
    cerebellum, 170
    cholinesterase inhibitors, 174
    cranial nerve VII, 164
    CT-guided abscess aspiration, 164
    discontinue ibuprofen, 162
    discriminative sensation, 170
    electrodiagnostic nerve conduction study, 166
    eye patch, 160
    facial nerve, 164
    fanning of toes, 162
    high-flow oxygen, 160
    hunter serotonin toxicity, 172
    incomplete spinal cord injury, 160
    intubation, 172
    isometric counterpressure, 164
    language, 174
    Lhermitte sign, 166

neurologic system (*continued*)
   middle meningeal artery, 166
   MRI of brain, 160, 162
   MRI of lumbar spine, 172
   neurodevelopmental evaluation, 170
   ocular lubricating ointment, 160
   skeletal survey radiographs, 166
   surgery, 160
   tension, 174
   triptans, 164
   vestibular rehabilitation, 164
neuromuscular junction, 164
neuropathy, 46
niacin, 22
Nikolsky sign, 32
nitrofurantoin-induced pulmonary injury, 204
nitroglycerin, 14
nonalcoholic fatty liver disease (NAFLD), 96
nondihydropyridine calcium channel
   blockers, 2
noninvasive screening test, 19
nonsteroidal anti-inflammatory drug
   (NSAID), 6, 52, 141, 146, 196, 226
norovirus, 246

obsessive compulsive disorder (OCD),
   168, 186
obstructive sleep apnea (OSA), 192
oculomotor nerve, 72
oligoclonal bands, 162
omalizumab, 206
omega-3 fatty acids, 4
ophthalmology, 76, 140
opioid, 190
oppositional defiant disorder (ODD), 178
optic neuritis, 68
oral candidiasis, 70
oral contraceptive pill (OCP), 233
oral decongestants, 74
oral dopamine agonists, 52
oral terbinafine, 40
organ procurement organization (OPO), 248
orlistat, 84
orthopnea, 4
orthostatic hypotension, 6
Ortolani tests, 140
Osgood-Schlatter disease, 140
osmotic demyelination syndrome (ODS), 220
osteoid osteomas, 142
osteomyelitis, 142
osteonecrosis, 155

osteoporosis, 85
otic antibiotic, 76
Ottawa ankle rules, 146
over-the-counter (OTC), 201
overweight, 50
oxytocin, 54

palpable purpura rash, 120, 224
pancreas, 90
pancreatic beta cells, 48
pancreatic enzyme replacement therapy
   (PERT), 84
panic disorder, 182
Papanicolaou (PAP) test, 231
papillary thyroid carcinoma, 56
paraganglioma, 6
paramyxovirus, 136
paraphimosis, 112
paraprotein, 114
parathyroid hormone (PTH), 49, 55
Parkinson's disease (PD), 160
paroxysmal nocturnal dyspnea (PND), 20
passive stretching, 154
Pasteurella multocida, 138
patent ductus arteriosus (PDA), 20
patient health questionnaire (PHQ-9), 186
PCR assay, 38
pectus excavatum, 144
pediatric urology, 108
pelvic inflammatory disease, 136
pelvic organ prolapse, 108
Penicillin, 122, 210
Penicillin G, 232
pentosan polysulfate, 106
peptic ulcer disease (PUD), 93, 97
percutaneous coronary intervention (PCI),
   10, 11, 12
perforated gastric ulcer, 94
performance anxiety, 183
pericardial effusion, 7
pericardial friction rub, 2
pericardiocentesis, 18
permanent pacemaker implantation, 16
permethrin, 30
permissive hypotension, 6
pernicious anemia, 115
persistent depressive disorder, 184
personal protective equipment (PPE), 246
Perthes disease, 146
pessary, 112
Peyronie's disease, 106

pharynx, 188
phenazopyridine, 106
phenylketonuria (PKU), 91
pheochromocytoma, 52
phimosis, 106
phlebitis, 16
phlebotomy, 122
phosphodiesterase-5 (PDE5) inhibitors, 104
pica, 122
pityriasis rosea, 40
pleuritis, 198
Pneumocystis jirovecii pneumonia (PJP), 134
pneumococcal polysaccharide (PPSV23)
    vaccine, 192
pneumothorax, 204
point-of-care ultrasound (POCUS), 132
point of maximal impulse (PMI), 23
polyarteritis nodosa (PAN), 150
polycystic kidney disease, 226
polycystic ovarian syndrome, 50
polymorphonuclear leukocyte (PMN), 93
polymyalgia rheumatica (PMR), 18
polysomnogram, 180
portal hypertension, 86
postcoital urinary voiding, 102
postconcussion syndrome, 174
postexposure prophylaxis (PEP), 129
postherpetic neuralgia, 136
post-traumatic stress disorder (PTSD), 8, 178
potassium, 14
Prader-Willi syndrome (PWS), 56
preeclampsia, 236
Prehn sign, 102
premature menarche, 60
premature ventricular contractions (PVCs), 5
premenstrual dysphoric disorder
    (PMDD), 190
priapism, 108
primary hyperparathyroidism, 104
primary sclerosing cholangitis (PSC), 84
Prinzmetal's variant angina (PVA), 20
professional practice
    abortion, 244
    blood transfusion, 248
    breastfeeding, 248
    burnout, 248
    cardiovascular, 244
    clinician impairment, 250
    contraception, 244
    decision-making, 246
    documentation, 246
emergency operations center, 246
epidemiology, 248
ethics committee, 250
gloved hands, 248
healthcare disparities, 244
hepatitis B, 248
hospital legal counsel, 244
immunization, 246
incident-to billing, 250
interprofessional, 248
late entry documentation, 250
living will, 244
mandated reporter, 244
medical error, 248
medicare, 250
optimal team practice, 244
physician-assisted death, 250
precision medicine, 250
professional interpreter, 250
sterilization, 244
surge capacity, 246
symptom control, 248
tail coverage, 246
washing hands, 250
propranolol, 164
proprotein convertase subtilisin/kexin type 9
    (PCSK9) inhibitor, 18
propylthiouracil (PTU), 46
prostate-specific antigen (PSA), 107, 108
prosthetic heart valve, 9
proton pump inhibitor (PPI), 86, 87, 92
Pseudomonas aeruginosa, 68
psoas sign, 82
psoriasis, 31, 32
psychiatry/behavioral science
    acute psychiatric emergency, 182
    adjustment disorder, 184
    beta-blockers, 184
    cluster B, 182
    dissociative amnesia, 188
    elderly male, 180
    elder neglect, 176
    empiric antibiotics, 186
    hypomanic episode, 176
    late luteal phase, 190
    lead toxicity, 178
    lipid panel, 176
    medication with food, 180
    MRI of brain, 180
    narcissistic, 178
    neuroleptic medications, 182

psychiatry/behavioral science (*continued*)
  pharmacological therapy, 178
  QT prolongation, 186
  reassurance, 186
  sleep hygiene, 184
  specific phobia, 188
  stimulants, 176
  weight gain, 182
pterygium, 66
pulmonary contusion, 206
pulmonary edema, 194
pulmonary system
  alpha-1-antitrypsin level, 194
  anterior axillary line, 202
  asthma, 210
  Barrel chest, 210
  carboxyhemoglobin saturation, 202
  chest physiotherapy, 200
  cigarette smoking, 194
  corticosteroids, 200
  croup, 200
  CT of chest, 198, 204, 210, 212
  currant jelly, 198
  D-dimer assay, 208
  decreased/absent tactile fremitus, 198
  digital clubbing, 206
  discolored sputum, 196
  drainage, 202
  endotracheal intubation, 206
  flail chest, 210
  fourth intercostal space, 202
  immunotherapy, 192
  inhalation chamber, 208
  LAIV, 208
  Light's criteria, 204
  macrolide, 202
  malignant mesothelioma, 200
  metastasis, 212
  NSAID, 196
  OTC cough, 202
  overnight polysomnography, 192
  peak flow meter, 202
  phrenic nerve compression, 206
  pulmonary embolism, 208
  pulmonary infection, 202
  refined ABCD assessment tool, 204
  right-sided cardiac catheterization, 212
  rigid bronchoscopy, 206
  sounds, 194
  sputum culture, 212
  status asthmaticus, 208

  surfactant, 192
  systemic corticosteroids, 198
  tension pneumothorax, 210
  thoracostomy tube, 192
  transudative effusion, 200
  wheeze, 210
pulse oximetry, 208
pulsus paradoxus, 16

QRS complex, 21
quinolones, 194

rabies immune globulin, 130
rabies vaccine, 130
radioiodine therapy, 48
Ranson criteria, 80
rash, 126
Raynaud's phenomenon, 149, 152
reactive arthritis, 148
reactive thrombocytosis, 148
reassurance, 6
rebound hypertension, 12
recombinant growth hormone, 56
Reed-Sternberg cells, 122
Reiter syndrome, 148
renal artery stenosis, 20, 216
renal system
  anticoagulation, 220
  asymptomatic abdominal mass, 224
  blood glucose, 218
  blood pressure, 222
  calcium gluconate, 222
  diabetes, 222
  dialysis, 224
  digoxin, 224
  ECG, 215
  edema, 216
  fluid resuscitation, 226
  hypertension, 222
  hypotension, 222
  IgA nephropathy, 214
  late-stage CKD 3, 214
  magnesium, 222
  metabolic acidosis, 218
  metabolic alkalosis, 226
  non-contrast computed tomography (CT), 224
  non-palpable, 226
  NSAID, 226
  pharynx and skin, 220
  phosphorus, 216

poststreptococcal glomerulonephritis, 220
potassium, 214, 216, 218
QT prolongation, 216
relieve obstruction, 216
renal artery stenosis, 216
tendinitis/tendon rupture, 218
ultrasound, 220
renin-angiotensin-aldosterone system
    (RAAS), 215
reproductive system (male/female)
    antiemetic, 228
    beta-hCG, 232
    breast ultrasound, 230
    CA-125, 234
    caffeine, 234
    cervical cerclage, 242
    cervical lesion, 240
    cesarean section, 228, 234
    Chadwick sign, 228
    Chandelier sign, 236
    contraception, 234
    corticosteroid, 242
    cystocele, 238
    endometriosis, 242
    estrogen/progesterone, 238
    forensic exam, 232
    full cervical dilation, 236
    hydatidiform mole, 230
    leopold maneuvers, 238
    linea nigra, 232
    mammograms, 228, 230
    menopause, 242
    nabothian cyst, 232
    Naegele's rule, 234
    ovarian torsion, 242
    placental abruption, 240
    premature rupture, 236
    reassurance, 236
    rectocele, 230
    shoulder dystocia, 228
    sun protection, 230
    Tanner stage II, 234
    TDap and influenza, 232
    transvaginal ultrasound, 238
    urgent delivery of fetus, 236
    uterine rupture, 228
residual volume (RV), 202
respiratory acidosis, 212
respiratory alkalosis, 218
respiratory syncytial virus (RSV), 192, 196
reticulocytes, 116

rhabdomyolysis, 22
rheumatic fever, 10
    acute, 28, 128
rheumatoid arthritis (RA), 119, 150
Rh immunoglobulin (RhIg), 240
rhinitis medicamentosa, 62
rhonchi, 204
rifaximin, 96
right sensorineural, 70
Rinne test, 69
rosacea, 30
rotavirus vaccine, 128

salmon-colored plaques, 31
Salter-Harris classification, 151
Salter-Harris (SH) IV fracture, 155
scabicide, 30
scabies, 29, 38
seborrheic keratosis (SK), 34
selective serotonin reuptake inhibitor
    (SSRI), 171, 180
serotonin norepinephrine reuptake inhibitors
    (SNRIs), 186
serum prolactin, 60
serum triglycerides, 34
sexually transmitted infection (STI), 137, 239
short-acting beta agonist (SABA), 197
shoulder immobilization, 154
sideroblastic anemia, 118
sinoatrial (SA) node, 2
sinus node dysfunction, 15
skeletal maturity, 152
skin biopsy, 29
slipped capital femoral epiphysis (SCFE), 158
small bowel obstruction (SBO), 100
smoking cessation, 32
sodium-glucose co-transporter 2 inhibitors
    (SGLT2), 54
soft-tissue lateral neck x-ray, 66
spinal cord injury (SCI), 173
spinal stenosis, 140
splenectomy, 92, 114
spondylolysis, 150
squamous cell carcinoma, 40, 94
stable angina, 24
Staphylococcus aureus, 64, 74, 94, 132, 234
stasis dermatitis, 15
ST-elevation myocardial infarction
    (STEMI), 9, 23
steroids, 70
Stevens-Johnson Syndrome (SJS), 34

Streptococcus pneumoniae, 198
Streptococcus pyogenes, 126
succussion splash, 98
sudden infant death syndrome (SIDS), 168
sulfonylureas, 56
sun protection factor (SPF), 33
superficial thrombophlebitis, 8
superior vena cava (SVC) syndrome, 208
surgical drainage, 80
surgical excision, 140
swan neck deformity, 154
syncope, risk of, 14
syndrome of inappropriate antidiuretic
     hormone (SIADH), 57
synthetic thyroxine, 48
Systemic Inflammatory Response System
     (SIRS), 127
systemic lupus erythematosus (SLE), 117, 139
systemic sclerosis, 152
systolic/diastolic pressures, 22

tachycardia, 92
tachypnea, 128
tardive dyskinesia, 82
temporal arteritis, 18
Tetralogy of Fallot (ToF), 18
thiamine, 80
thiazolidinediones (TZDs), 50
Thompson test, 154
thoracentesis, 198
thoracic aortic aneurysm, 25
thoracic outlet syndrome, 158
thoracolumbar-sacral orthosis (TLSO), 156
thrombophilia screen, 72
thrombotic thrombocytopenic purpura
     (TTP), 121
thumb spica splint immobilization, 152
Tietze syndrome, 26
tinea pedis, 34
Tinel test, 156
toddler fracture, 148
tonsillar abscess, 72
tophi, 74
topical antibiotics, 71, 132
topical corticosteroids, 30, 40, 76
topical immunomodulator, 136
Torsades de pointes, 16
torus palatinus, 66
total lung capacity (TLC), 201
tourette syndrome (TS), 168
toxoplasmosis, 126

transesophageal echocardiogram (TEE), 16, 20
transitional cell carcinoma, 104
trauma-focused psychotherapy, 176
traumatic hyphema, 68
trephination, 142
trichobezoar, 90
Trichophyton rubrum, 33
trichotillomania, 182
tricuspid stenosis, 7
trimethoprim/sulfamethoxazole (TMP-SMX),
     110, 134
triplane, 156
troponin I, 10
Trousseau's sign, 48
Turner syndrome, 17
T waves, 1
tympanic membrane (TM), 65
tympanogram, 66
tyrosine kinase inhibitor (TKI), 118

ulcerative colitis, 98
ultrasound, 6
  abdominal, 83
  breast, 230
  cardiovascular system, 6
  color doppler, 104
  endocrine system, 43
  gallbladder polyps, 79
  gastrointestinal system, 98
  liver, 96
  nutrition, 98
  pelvic, 237
  renal, 215, 220
  transvaginal, 238
uremic syndrome, 224
urethroplasty, 110
urinalysis, 109
urinary alkalization, 82
urinary tract infection (UTI), 53, 109, 226
urothelial cell carcinoma, 104
uterine atony, 240
uterine leiomyoma, 240

vancomycin, 90
varicella-zoster virus (VZV) syndrome, 42
varicocele, 108
varicose vein sclerotherapy, 15
vasodilators, 86
vasopressin, 54
vasopressors, 23
vasospastic angina, 20

vasovagal, 10
venous thromboembolism, 120
ventilation-perfusion (V/Q) scan, 196
ventricular fibrillation, 12, 23
ventricular septal defect (VSD), 4
vestibular labyrinthitis, 76
vestibular schwannomas, 74
viral etiology, 74
vital capacity (VC), 201
vitamin B, 78
vitamin B12, 82, 118
vitamin C, 118
vitamin D, 44
vitamin K, 124
vitiligo, 30
voiding cystourethrogram (VCUG), 110
von Willebrand disease (VWD), 117, 122

warfarin therapy, 19
water hammer pulse, 26
weight management, 32
Wernicke-Korsakoff syndrome, 79
white blood cells (WBC), 104, 121
Wilms tumor, 214
Wilson disease, 68
Wolff-Parkinson-White Syndrome, 22

xanthelasma, 44

yellow fever, 246

zoledronic acid, 88
Zollinger-Ellison Syndrome (ZES), 94